# LEARNING DISABLED CHILDREN GROWING UP
## A follow-up into adulthood

# LEARNING DISABLED CHILDREN GROWING UP

## A follow-up into adulthood

Otfried Spreen

Department of Psychology
University of Victoria, Canada

Oxford      New York
Oxford University Press
1988

**Library of Congress Cataloging-in-Publication Data**

Spreen, Otfried.
   Learning disabled children growing up.

   Bibliography: p.
   Includes index.
   1. Learning disabilities--Longitudinal studies.
2. Learning disabled children--Longitudinal studies.
I. Title. [DNLM: 1. Follow-Up Studies. 2. Learning
Disorders. WS 110 S768L]
RJ506.L4S67 1988      362.1'96855     87-28171
ISBN 0-19-520641-X

© 1987 by Swets & Zeitlinger

Published in 1987 by
Swets & Zeitlinger bv
Heereweg 347
2161 CA Lisse
The Netherlands

Published in 1988 in the United States by
Oxford University Press, Inc.
200 Madison Avenue, New York, New York 10016

Oxford is a registered trademark of Oxford University Press

ISBN (U.S.) 520641-X

Printing (last digit): 987654321

# TABLE OF CONTENTS

## Acknowledgement

The support of the first Phase of this study by Health and Welfare Canada (Grant 610-1034-29) and for the major part of the second part of the project by the Medical Research Council of Canada (Grant MA-6972) and the support for the expansion of the study by the B.C. Health Care Research Foundation (1981/2) is gratefully acknowledged. Additional support came from the University of Victoria Research Committee, and from the Ministry of Labor, Government of British Columbia (Summer Student Employment Programme). This study was facilitated by short term study leaves granted to the principal investigator in 1981 and 1985 by the University of Victoria.

I would like to thank Adele Hern for coordinating the second Phase of the follow-up and conducting the interviews; Charles Simpson for contributing neurological examinations for all our subjects; and Thirell Murphy for doing most of the test examinations. Phase I interviews were conducted by Sharolyn Langhout, Jae Ranschaert and Giselda Evans-Cockle, and the data entry organized by Jane Brett. Additional testing, data coding, and analyses were done by Joanne Lavergne, Karen Salter, Sonya Spreen, Bryan Talarico and Sherry Williamson. Iryna Black, Barbara Burnside, Robert Haaf, Adele Hern, Shelly O'Connor, Vivian Russell, Karen Salter and Francine Sarazin provided analyses of sections of the information collected in this study.

Special thanks for many valuable comments on the manuscript go to Dirk Bakker, Bill Gaddes, Georgia Spreen, and particularly to Klaus Plasterk of Swets & Zeitlinger for his careful editorial reading.

Most of all, our thanks to the participants in the study for their interest, their willingness to share their experiences with us and to donate a considerable amount of their time. We hope that these results will contribute to improved attention to future learning-disabled children during their formative years in school.

# Introduction

Constancy and change are the main themes of current research in human development. Brim and Kagan (1980) point out that Western thinking has led to the expectation of connectivity, to hereditary and environmental determinism, and hence to continuity of development. Yet the evidence presented in this remarkable book demonstrates continuity only to a very limited extent: variations in behaviour during infancy show only very limited predictive validity for reaction patterns in the distant future, often accounting for as little as 2 to 8 percent of the variance. While such limited evidence for constancy becomes more reliable in middle childhood, Brim and Kagan note that higher constancy is mainly based on measures related to the 'biological organization of language ability' (vocabulary) as well as the stability of the environment.

In a wider sense, the study to be reported here investigates constancy and change in groups of learning-disabled children as they grow into adulthood, and compares them to average learners. The presupposition of connectedness would lead to the assumption that the rank-ordering of subjects' abilities will be maintained in most areas, especially in the domain of physical deficits and health. Yet, as Starfield and Pless (1980) have shown, considerable changes occur in the individual between age 2 and 10, even for neurosensory problems and convulsions. New patterns of behaviour appear to replace old ones. Stein and Dawson (1980) conclude that so many variables affect the outcome of central nervous system damage that no single explanation is capable of explaining what constitutes recovery: growth and regeneration of nerve fibers, activation of 'latent synapses', release from 'diaschisis' (recovery from shock in otherwise healthy brain areas), denervation supersensitivity (formation of new synaptic connections of remaining fibers), vicarious takeover of function by other brain areas and multiple control, as well as behavioural response substitution. If constancy and change are so poorly delineated in the neurological and health area, long-term development of behaviour is even more likely to be subject to change. In fact, investigating change rather than continuity, and finding satisfactory explanatory models for both, seems to be the most important problem facing developmental psychology today. This monograph may provide some facts in a limited area of investigation to assist in this goal.

The primary objective of the project described in this monograph was to obtain comprehensive information about the long-term adjustment of learning-disabled children on a prospective basis. As the following review of the literature shows, only a few studies have addressed this question, providing only partial answers; some previous studies also include rather misleading conclusions based on retrospective reviews of groups already identified as deviant (e.g., convicted juvenile offenders). Virtually no information is available on health adjustment, changes in neurological or neuropsychological status or occupational adjustment, income, and social adjustment of formerly learning-disabled children as they reach adulthood.

The first part of this study (Spreen 1978a, 1983) (Phase I) followed 203 learning-disabled (LD) children up to the mean age of 18 years in 1977, and was based primarily on structured interview, questionnaire, and school record data. This provided a unique data base to (a) continue the follow-up to a median age of 25 (mean 24.37) years (Phase II); (b) to assess changes in neurological status by reexamination and comparison with the original neurological examinations conducted between the ages of 8 and 12 years; (c) to assess the neuropsychological status changes by reexamination and comparison with previous test results obtained at the time of the original referral when our clients were between 8 and 12 years old; (d) to examine whether the original subdivision of our sample of LD children into a group with definite neurological impairment, a group with minimal (or questionable) impairment, and a group without neurological impairment was of any significance for the long-term outcome, and whether any one or all LD groups differed from a carefully chosen control group of 52 'average learners'.

The specific objectives of the project were (a) to develop long-term data for the major portion of the sample who participated in Phase I and II; (b) to provide an objective data base for well-reasoned predictions about the future of children with learning disabilities in general, and with specific patterns of educational and neurological impairment in particular; (c) to review the educational remediation and medical treatment which our participants had received with a view towards possible recommendations for future clients, school authorities and medical practitioners (e.g. the effectiveness of learning assistance classes or of stimulant drug therapy as compared to other forms of intervention). However, it is recognized that our project did not provide rigorously controlled treatment groups.

A clarification of the usage of the term 'learning disability' (LD) may be in order. In North-American usage the term frequently refers inclusively to all children (and adults) with learning problems. British (Rutter 1978) and German (Nissen 1980) authors usually distinguish between 'learning backwardness' or 'learning handicap' and 'learning disorder' ,'specific' or 'partial' learning disability, the former referring to children with borderline intelligence (IQ 70 to 85 or 70 to 89) and the latter to children with intelligence in the average range ($> 85$ or $> 89$). It should be stressed that, although our original selection criteria included all participants with IQs of 70 or higher, the majority of the subjects had IQs of 85 or better. This question is more specifically addressed later by special analyses with restricted and matched IQ samples.

This volume presents specific data on each of the many variables of interest. The reader may also wish to consult the book for the normative data derived from our control group of normal learners at the ages of 19 and 25, including a number of neuropsychological tests for which norms are not yet available.

# Review of the Literature

A detailed review of the pertinent literature was presented by Helper (1980) and Spreen (1981). The following summary will only briefly deal with questions of definition and prevalence of learning disability and with the existing follow-up research of LD children in general and of LD children with indications of brain damage in particular. Other studies will be referred to in the context of the description of our results.

There is little doubt that children with LD have been a source of increasing concern for educators, psychologists, physicians, and most of all for parents. Legislators and numerous commissions and associations have been involved because of the social, educational, and financial implications of helping and dealing with LD children (CELDIC 1970; Clements 1966; Clements & Peters 1963; Cruickshank 1979; Myklebust 1973; National Advisory Committee 1968). Numerous different terms and definitions have been used, primarily dependent on the discipline and philosophy of the investigator, and ranging from highly inclusive to very restrictive (Gaddes 1976). Cruickshank (1977) provides an example of the more inclusive definitions, viewing LD as: '(1) a problem of acquisition of developmental skills, academic achievement, social adjustment and secondarily emotional growth and development; (2) which may be of any etiological origin; (3) may be observed in children and youth of any age; and (4) of any intellectual level of function'. Cruickshank docs, however, indicate his own restrictive bias by including in his definition that LDs 'are the result of perceptual processing deficits which in turn may be the result of (diagnosed or inferred) neurophysiological dysfunction occurring at prenatal, perinatal or (in the case of linguistic dysfunction) at postnatal periods of development'. A more restrictive definition is supported by Rutter (1978) and by Bateman and Schiefelbusch (1969) who require 'a discrepancy between measures of intellectual, cognitive and academic potential and current level of performance; dysfunction in the learning process; and absence of other primary factors such as mental retardation, cultural, sensory and/or educational inadequacy; or serious emotional disturbance'.

In addition to the general definition of LD, numerous types of LD, usually referred to as 'specific LD' (Bakker & Satz 1970) have been developed, usually singling out specific reading disability (as opposed to general 'backwardness' , Yule 1973) as a special group.

5

Prevalence rates of LD vary widely, mainly because of differences in definition, but tend to range from 5 to 15 percent of the school population (Gaddes 1976). Approximately half of this population has been described as having evidence of brain damage of varying degree (Minskoff 1973; Myklebust et al. 1969; Page-El and Grossman 1973; Rubin and Balow 1971; Silverman and Metz 1973). Many authors stress, however, that the presence of brain damage should not be interpreted as a direct causal factor since the interaction between even mild degrees of deviance, social factors, and educational expectations may lead to continued failure experiences, discouragement, and attitude change. Such interactions, combined with educational labelling may even lead to self-fulfilling prophecies about the outcome of LD (Bryan & Bryan 1975). Nevertheless, brain dysfunction as a contributing factor in the development of many LD children has been recognized by a majority of authors (Birch 1964; Boll & Reitan 1972; Chall & Mirsky 1978; Cruickshank 1971; de la Cruz et al. 1973; Deutsch & Schumer 1970; Gesell & Armatruda 1947; Helper 1980; Isaacson 1968; Johnson & Myklebust 1967; Kaspar et al. 1971; Rutter et al. 1970a; Wender 1971).

Due to the nature of educational, medical, and psychological counseling, diagnostic inferences of brain dysfunction as a contributing cause of LD are usually made on the basis of short observation and examination periods. Detailed educational or other treatment prescriptions are frequently given, but the results of such treatments become known to the counseling professional only if the child returns for further assistance. Similarly, while the validity of some of the indicators of brain dysfunction may be checked by correlational validation procedures, the persistence of these indicators during the further development of the individual remains unknown. Follow-up studies of newborns with indications of brain damage at birth suggest that a large proportion of 'at risk' babies are completely normal and free of symptoms at age 3 or 7 (Graham et al. 1962, 1963; Nichols & Chen 1981; Ondarza-Landwehr 1979), but such expectations are not necessarily true for children diagnosed as brain damaged at a later age.

Only a limited number of studies have attempted a long-term follow-up of children with LD. Most of these studies are concerned with special groups of children, i.e. hyperkinetic, autistic, speech and perceptual handicaps, emotional or behavioural adjustment problems, or with the specific effects of treatment. Other studies focused on the vocational outcome of LD with somewhat contradictory results to be discussed in Section 8.

One recent study (Bruck 1985) may serve as an example of LD follow-up studies. This study, though comprehensive in nature, deliberately omitted the dimension of neurological impairment, and excluded children with IQ scores less than 90, primary behavioural or emotional disturbances, major neurological abnormalities or physical disabilities from a Montreal clinic-referred file sample. As a result, the LD in these subjects was probably milder than in most other samples. Only 101 out of a total of 259 subjects participated in the study. All had been referred because of LD, but no specific cut-off procedure or definition was used. The author established a peer control group (friends or relatives of the participants without learning problems) and a second control group of 51 siblings without learning problems. The second control group was chosen because the peer control group tended to include too many 'atypically achievement oriented and successful' subjects in 'both academic and occupational domains'. The follow up from an age of 5 to 10 years to the age of 17 to 29 showed only minimal ( and mostly statistically nonsignificant) differences from the sibling control group, but substantial differences from the peer control group in employment rates, occupational levels, and asocial behaviour, although LD females had more adjustment problems than controls. Bruck concludes that 'LD subjects were not underemployed, ...not at risk for becoming high school dropouts, ...did go on to higher education,... although all LD students reported mild to moderate difficulties with their academic studies' (pg.125). Bruck also found 'no association between juvenile delinquency, problems of drug and alcohol abuse, and childhood learning disabilities', although they 'were at risk to show problems in the area of peer relationships and psychological adjustment,...in the absence of extreme forms of deviance'(pg.126). The author concludes that 'LD indi- viduals lead well adjusted and productive lives'(pg.126). These optimistic conclusions may be partly due to the exclusion of more serious, clearly defined LDs, the choice of a sibling control group rather than an average learner group representative for the referral area, and the fact that LDs and controls were equated for number of years of education (a potentially fruitful research variable), as well as the wide age range (mean age at follow-up 21 years) which tends to increase variance even though an attempt to reduce this by breakdown into 'in-school - out-of-school' subjects, and by covariance analysis was made.

Follow-up studies pose considerable methodological problems. Schon- haut and Satz (1983), in a review of 17 follow-up studies of LD children, considered the following criteria to be critical: (a) an adequate follow-up period; (b) a sufficiently large sample size; (c) a satisfactory method of sample selection; (d) an adequate comparison group; (e) a valid and objective measure of reading or learning disability. Although none of the 17 studies met all criteria satisfactorily, studies by Howden (1967), Rawson (1968), Rutter, Graham and Yule (1970), Satz et al. (1978) and Spreen (1978) were considered acceptable. From their review the authors conclud- ed that the prognosis for academic success in LD children is extremely poor, with the exception of children from families with high socio- economic status (SES) and of children involved in intensive rehabilitation programs. LD children were found to be more likely to drop out of school, and unlikely to obtain jobs requiring high school completion. Little is known about the occupational choice, job satisfaction, social and emotional adjustment, or the benefits of early diagnosis and educational and medical treatment. The authors conclude that prognosis is poor in the few areas which have been studied, but that large areas of adjustment have not been covered as yet. They did not review specific studies of brain-damaged or hyperactive children because of problems in clearly defining these terms. However, in the context of the current research it is important to consider some of this research.

The concept of brain damage or 'minimal brain dysfunction' as a major cause of learning disability has been popular since Strauss' first books on the subject (Strauss & Kephart 1955; Strauss & Lehtinen 1947). The concept was reinforced by the influential study of a 'continuum of reproductive casualty' by Pasamanick and Knobloch (1960). More recently, detailed explorations of the etiology and the early developmental problems of such children have been presented by Broman et al. (1975) and Nichols and Chen (1981). The term is frequently used also during the school age period and has been the topic of several conferences and books (de la Cruz et al. 1973, Satz & Fletcher 1980, Tarnopol & Tarnopol 1977). However, all through its existence, the concept has been severely criticized on the grounds that it merely provides labelling and encourages educational resignation rather than providing a useful rationale for education and treatment. Another frequent criticism is that there is no agreement on the symptoms needed to define the condition, and that, while the term would seem to refer to a medical (physical) diagnosis, the symptoms most often described are behavioural or 'soft' neurological signs which may be maturational in nature, unreliable, or difficult to elicit during the neurological examination (Rutter 1982). In a book on minimal brain dysfunction, Helper (1980) reviewed studies which followed children with this diagnosis. Although acknowledging that many of the published studies are fraught with methodological problems, Helper concludes that these children 'will have a high risk of some lasting deficits in functioning' (pg. 110), especially of repeating grades in school, and, if the child is hyperactive, 'an elevated risk of antisocial behaviour'. Beyond these very broad conclusions, he stated that 'outcomes depend on the nature and extent of cognitive and behavioural manifestations of MBD, the child's general intellectual level, and perhaps on his SES and family'.

Examples of specific studies include the work of Rubin and Balow (1971) who followed kindergarten children for a period of 4 years and found that 41 % of the children still had serious learning problems in spite of normal measures of language, intelligence and school readiness at age 5. Denhoff (1973) mentioned in his follow-up of infant to preschool age children over a 10-year period that they often showed a changing clinical picture 'with diminishing signs of neurological dysfunction and evidence of increasing

IQ scores'(pg.204). Dykman et al. (1973) reported on 53 14-year old returnees who had originally been tested and reported to have MBD as compared to 22 control subjects. The authors found that low IQ scores were predictors of poor academic progress and that many of their subjects suffered from poor self-image and dislike of school. While Koppitz (1971) found no relationship between neurological dysfunction and follow-up achievement, Johnson and Neumann (1975) noted some improvement over a 7-year period, but less improvement if the IQ was low, the EEG was abnormal, or if psychiatric disorder was present in childhood. Laufer (1971) and Kleinpeter and Goellnitz (1976) found an increase in educational and psychiatric problems over a period of 10 to 12 years. Gottesman (1975, 1979) also reported persisting reading problems, but diminishing neurological signs. Similar results were presented by Ackerman, Dykman, and Peters (1977a).

The 10-year follow-up conducted on children diagnosed as having cerebral dysfunction by Kaste (1972) is one of four unpublished dissertations on follow-up research and one of the most comprehensive studies to date. Kaste studied three groups of children with varying degrees of brain dysfunction along with a control group with no evidence of cerebral dysfunction. One major problem of this study was that the control group was comprised of children who had behaviour problems severe enough to warrant referral to a pediatric clinic. In general, one half of her subjects continued to have serious adjustment problems, although there were no statistical differences between the four groups in the adjustment ratings. In particular, members of the groups exhibiting the most severe dysfunction remained poorly controlled and poorly coordinated individuals who were generally inadequate according to societal standards.

A recently published study by Herbst and Roesler (1986) presents one of the most detailed follow-up of children with congenital brain damage to date. While the total sample of 230 participants included groups of mildly and moderately retarded, the subsample of 58 subjects with IQs between 70 and 119 (mean 95.66) is comparable to the present study. At a mean age of 12, this sample showed neurological abnormalities in 14.9%, EEG abnormalities in 55.3%, and abnormal x-ray findings in 42.5% of the subjects. Etiology was primarily described as 'developmental delay, and abnormal factors of delivery. The sample was studied at a mean age of 22, using a battery of intelligence, motor, concentration, and the draw-a-man test as well as a neurological reexamination and a structured interview. The authors examined factors of social environment as well as biological factors, and related both to occupational, social, personal adjustment and delinquency. A normal control group of 18 subjects was compared to 18 of the participants matched for IQ. Individual results from this East German study will be referred to in the appropriate sections. However, the general findings indicate severe disadvantage in schooling and occupational

9

achievement for this group, as well as continuing neurological abnormalities, poorer social adjustment and higher delinquency rates.

A recent review of the adult developmental perspective of LD (Polloway et al. 1984) stresses a life-span developmental approach: what appears as transitory academic problems in school, may change not only in complexity, but may also extend into many other areas of adjustment as the adult faces increasing societal demands on emotional maturity, acceptable social behaviour, vocational competence, and self-direction. For these reasons, the study to be presented here attempted a comprehensive approach, including not only the investigation of problems directly related to school learning, but including most areas of adult adjustment.

# A. METHOD

## 1. Subjects

The files of the Neuropsychology Laboratory, University of Victoria, and of the Special Counsellor's Office, Nanaimo School District No.68 were screened for all children referred for learning-problem between 1966 and 1972 who were between 8 and 12 years of age at that time. Further requirements for inclusion in the first phase of the study were that a minimum of 4 years had elapsed between initial testing and follow-up and that a neurological examination had been conducted. As Table 1 1 shows, a total of 303 of these children were traced and 255 participated either in the Phase I subject or parent interview or both, a participation rate of 84%. Phase I used a catchup prospective design (Harway, Mednick, & Mednick 1984).

The LD subjects were broken down into three groups on the basis of the neurological examination (evaluated by a uniform coding system, see Appendix 5). Group 1 (BD) consisted of subjects with 'hard' neurological signs, containing 64 subjects. The 82 subjects in group 2 (MBD) had only 'soft' neurological signs, and the 57 subjects of Group 3 (LD) had no neurological findings. All subjects were traced to their present addresses and contacted. Subjects whose present addresses were untraceable or who had moved out of the Vancouver Island or Lower Mainland (Vancouver and area) regions were dropped from the study. Only two subjects refused to participate.

In addition to the LD children, a control group of 52 subjects was selected from two senior secondary and one junior secondary school in the Greater Victoria School District. Teachers were asked to select a random sample of students who, between the age of 8 to 12, had experienced no learning problems nor exceptionally good progress. These criteria were verified during the follow-up interview and participants who did not meet them were rejected from the study. The control group was matched with the LD group for median age, sex, and handedness at the time of the original referral. They were also chosen from neighbourhoods with similar socio-economic status and matched for the occupational and educational level of their parents. Of an initial 67 control subjects, 52 remained after matching. Only one subject refused to participate.

For part of the analysis of the Phase I results, 48 LD subjects were dropped, because their IQ at the time of the initial assessment indicated that they fell into the mentally handicapped range (below 70), because they were referred primarily because of emotional disorders, or because they had acquired brain damage at some time during childhood. Some of the Phase I results will be presented both for the full groups and for the reduced groups. In addition, for some analyses (educational achievement) the sample was further restricted to subjects with an IQ > 90.

A review of scores on the Wide Range Achievement Test (WRAT) at referral age confirmed that 95% of the children were 1 *SD* or more below the expected grade level on reading, spelling or arithmetic as compared to local norms (McAllister & Spreen 1981). Local norms were used rather than test manual norms, since the normative data study showed considerably higher achievement in regional public schools than indicated in the 1978 test manual (similar differences have been reported in other Western Canadian cities).

In Phase II of the study, all subjects who had participated in Phase I, with the exception of the 48 subjects dropped for the reasons mentioned above, were included and contact attempted. Table 1-1 shows the breakdown of the subject search and the final number of subjects. This part of the study follows a real-time prospective design.

*Table 1-1: Subjects Participating in Phase I and II*

Phase I (Mean age 18; average period following initial testing 8 years)

|  | Group 1 | Group 2 | Group 3 | Controls | Total |
|---|---|---|---|---|---|
| Traced |  |  |  | 303 |  |
| Participated | 64 | 82 | 57 | 52 | 255 |
| Subject participated |  |  |  | 216 |  |
| Parent participated |  |  |  | 248 |  |
| Untraceable, died, refused |  |  |  | 48 |  |
| Excluded* |  |  |  | 48 |  |
| Reduced *n* | 52 | 69 | 34 | 52 | 207 |
| Mean Age at Referral | 9.7 | 9.8 | 9.9 |  |  |
| Mean Age at Phase I | 18.7 | 18.9 | 18.5 |  |  |

Phase II (Mean age 25; average period following initial test 15 years)

|  | LD | % | Controls | % | Total | % |
|---|---|---|---|---|---|---|
| Phase I subjects |  |  |  |  |  |  |
| traced | 148 |  | 51 |  | 199 |  |
| participated | 119 | 80 | 46 | 90 | 165 | 82 |
| refused** | 19 |  | 3 |  | 22 |  |
| deceased | 4 |  | - |  | 4 |  |
| untraceable | 4 |  | 1 |  | 5 |  |

12

*Table 1 continued*

| | | | | | | |
|---|---|---|---|---|---|---|
| lived too far away | 2 | | 1 | | 3 | |
| total lost | 29 | | 5 | | 34 | |
| **additional subjects** | | | | | | |
| traced | 32 | | 5 | | 37 | |
| participated | 22 | 69 | 5 | 100 | 27 | 73 |
| refused** | 6 | | - | | 6 | |
| too far away | 4 | | - | | 4 | |
| total lost | 10 | | - | | 10 | |
| **total sample** | | | | | | |
| traced | 180 | | 56 | | 236 | |
| participated | 141 | 78 | 51 | 91 | 192 | 81 |
| refused | 25 | | 3 | | 28 | |
| untraced | 6 | | 1 | | 7 | |
| deceased | 4 | | - | | 4 | |
| too far away | 4 | | 1 | | 5 | |
| **available for Phase II** | | | | | | |
| interview | 140 | | 51 | | 191 | |
| tests | 136 | | 51 | | 187 | |
| MMPI (total) | 113 | | 47 | | 160 | |
| MMPI (excluding invalid profiles) | | | | | 153 | |
| neurological re-examination | 126 | | 47 | | 173 | |
| Mean age at first referral | 9.9 | | 9.8 | | 9.9 | |
| Mean age at Phase II follow-up | 24.4 | | 24.1 | | 24.2 | |

Breakdown into Group Membership of Participants in Phase II:

| | | male | female |
|---|---|---|---|
| Group 1 | 67 | 47 | 20 |
| Group 2 | 73 | 55 | 18 |
| Group 3 | 35 | 25 | 10 |
| Group 4 | 51 | 31 | 20 |
| | 226 | 158 | 68 |

* excluding subjects with IQs less than 70, with brain damage acquired during childhood, and with primary emotional disorders.

** reasons for refusal: didn't like last interview 3, personal reasons 3, alcoholic in centre 1, doing fine 1, not interested 7, missed several appointments and did not return calls 4.

Additional subjects added to the study were mainly from the original subject pool who had refused to participate in Phase I, but who were willing to participate in Phase II when contacted again. This may explain the relatively high refusal rate in Table 1-1 for this group.

The total sample represented all cases of the Neuropsychology Clinic with complete records on file within the ranges of age and intelligence specified, excluding subjects with brain damage acquired during childhood, and with primary emotional disorder. Hence, it is representative of our clinic population. It should be noted that, in terms of academic ability or disability pattern, the sample also did not differ from an unselected independent sample of 309 8- to 13-year-old LD children referred to the Greater Victoria School Board Learning Assistance Centre. In both samples, only 9 % of the children had a specific reading or spelling disability and 7 % had a specific arithmetic disability defined as more than 1 $SD$ below the regional mean with spelling and reading within one $SD$. The cognitive abilities of the School Board sample (defined as verbal, spatial and memory abilities measured with the WISC or WISC-R) were slightly better than in our sample but the difference was not significant (Tuokko 1982). The male: female ratio was 2.3:1 , and does not differ significantly from that reported in other studies (Finucci & Childs 1981). Hence, we are confident that the sample of this follow-up project is reasonably representative of LD children in the Greater Victoria communities, a Western Canadian city with a population of 220,000, and adjacent semi-rural areas.

A comparison of the IQ scores at the time of the initial referral of subjects participating in Phase II and those who were lost from the study is shown in Table 1-2.

*Table 1-2: IQ-Scores at Time of Original Referral for Participating and Nonparticipating Subjects in Phase II Recall by Group.*

|  | 1 | 2 | 3 | All 3 Groups |
|---|---|---|---|---|
| Nonparticip. | 99.00 | 106.82 | 106.38 | 104.18 |
| $n$ | ( 9) | ( 11) | ( 8) | ( 28) |
| Participants | 87.94 | 94.84 | 102.21 | 93.53 |
| $n$ | ( 51) | ( 58) | ( 24) | ( 133) |

| Participants/Nonparticipants | $F = 10.67, p < .001$ |
|---|---|
| Group | $F = 9.09, p < .001$ |

The scores of participating subjects were significantly lower than for those not participating in all three LD groups, although no significant group by participation interaction was found. The reason for this difference can only be inferred from our conversation with those subjects who were traced, but

14

who refused participation. For the most part, these former LD clients did not wish to be reminded of their school experiences, said that they were doing alright or could not find the time to participate. It would seem that the selective dropout from the study reflects that these somewhat brighter subjects were perhaps more sensitive to the follow-up questions, had less need for or even a fear of being viewed as 'LD' subjects again, while those participating were perhaps the more severely impaired subjects who still had a need to discuss their experiences and possibly receive some psychological support through the interview and testing. It should be noted that the difference between participants and nonparticipants at the time of referral was restricted to IQ tests. A multivariate comparison of the two groups on other tests was not significant.

Selective attrition of this type raises the question, however, how severely the results of the study are affected by IQ differences, since the groups after attrition differed significantly on this measure. An attempt was made to answer this question by repeating some of the analyses using IQ-matched groups (as well as by means of stepwise regression and covariance) throughout the results sections and will be addressed in Section 24.

**2.The Initial Referral, Information and Tests.**

The following information was available as predictor variables for the three LD groups:

a) The results of the neurological examination between the ages of 8 and 12.

b) Group membership as described above.

c) Results of a battery of neuropsychological tests given at the time of the initial referral, including intelligence and school achievement tests. The specific neuropsychological tests included the Embedded Figures Test, the Halstead Category Test, the Benton Stereognosis Test, the Sentence Repetition Test, the Trail Making Test, the Dynamic Visual Retention Test, the Benton Visual Retention Test, a Lateral Dominance Examination, the Tactual Performance Test, the Finger Tapping Test, Writing Time of name for right and left hand, Hand Grip Strength, Sound Recognition, Tonal Memory, Right-Left Orientation, and an Aphasia Screening Test. Several subtest scores on these tests are also available.

d) Basic descriptive information at the time of referral (sex, age, handedness, educational level and occupation of the parents).

It should be noted here that the three groups of LD children at the time of initial referral differed slightly but significantly on measures of intelligence (Verbal IQs 88.9, 94.4, and 99.8 respectively). On retest at the time of follow-up Phase II, the respective scores were 85.3, 88.4, and 90.8. The Performance IQ scores at time I were 88.5, 96.7, and 101.9 respectively; at time II these scores changed to 83.5, 91.9, and 92.6. The time difference was

15

significant, but group by time interaction effects were not. It should be remembered that the WAIS-R produces scores generally 5 to 6 points lower than the WISC (which was given to a majority of our subjects at the time of referral) (Matarazzo 1972). Hence the time difference is probably an artifact. Nevertheless, the group difference should be kept in mind during the analysis of the outcome data (see also Section 15 and 24 of this report).

### 3. Follow-up Phase I

All subjects were contacted by letter, followed by a phone call arranging a specific interview date. Three principal interviewers and two additional interviewers conducted the interview at the convenience of the participants and their parents, either at the University of Victoria or at home or at another place of their choice. The majority of the interviews were conducted at the home of the participants. Because the control group lived mainly in the Victoria area, more interviews with this group were conducted on the University campus. Subjects living in institutions (psychiatric, prison) were interviewed at a suitable location of the institution. Interviews in all four groups were conducted in random order so that relative experience of the interviewer did not selectively affect group differences. Interviewers were not aware of the interviewee's assignment to any of the groups. Interviews with the parent and the participant were always conducted by different interviewers to avoid carry-over from one interview to the other; this also made it impossible to inform either the parents or the participant of the answers given by the other party (as was frequently requested).

The following follow-up information was obtained during Phase I of the study:

a) a structured personal interview covering 163 items of personal, emotional, educational, occupational adjustment and history (Appendix 2).

b) an identical interview, conducted separately and by a different interviewer with one or both of the parents.

c) The Permanent School Record Card information, obtained from the last school attended (or the school board offices) with permission of the participant and the parent.

d) A behaviour rating scale filled in by the parent, consisting of 30 6-point ratings on major bipolar adjectives describing the participant.

e)The Personal Adjustment Inventory (Bell 1962) including 140 yes/no questions answered by the participant and covering the home, health, social and personal/emotional adjustment areas.

f) A 12 item rating of the participant's behaviour during the interview made by the interviewer after completion of the interview (Appendix 3).

## 4. Follow-up Phase II

All subjects were traced and contacted by letter at their present address, followed by a phone call, requesting their collaboration and setting up an appointment, if they were willing and able to participate. Subjects who worked during the day or who lived outside of the Greater Victoria area were given appointments during evening hours or on Saturdays or at a time when they would be visiting Victoria. In some cases, the Phase II study was conducted in other towns. Subjects were reimbursed for travel expenses, lunch, and lost wages if the appointment could not be made on a day off work.

The general format of the Phase II follow-up included a neurological examination at the neurologist's office in the morning, followed by approximately five hours at the University Laboratory, including an interview which lasted between 40 and 60 minutes, and three and one half to four hours of neuropsychological testing. A personality questionnaire was filled out last, and frequently completed at the home of the participant and mailed back.

Many subjects requested information about the results of the tests. This was provided by the principal investigator or his associate after the session or at a separate appointment, or by letter. The information was provided in a brief but encouraging manner, and frequently included comments on topics of special concern to the participant if appropriate. Occasionally, a meeting with concerned parents (with permission of the participant) was also included in the follow-up.

The neurological examination followed a standard format (Appendix 5). The checklist is loosely based on the routine clinical neurological examination and serves to objectify the findings. The neurologist did not know what neurological findings, if any, had been obtained at the first referral neurological examination and did not take a health history in order to remain 'blind' as to the group membership of a given participant. Only in a few cases were participants recognized as former patients, and in some cases group placement was evident because of obvious neurological impairment. In one case, the neurological examination was conducted in another city by another neurologist who was instructed in the use of the checklist by the project neurologist. The 93-item interview also used a standard format (Appendix 4) although the participants were given sufficient time to discuss a given topic in more detail if they wished. The tests (Appendix 1) were administered in standard format following the respective manuals. The personality questionnaire (MMPI) was given in standard form, although some participants with poor reading ability were allowed to use the taped version; if taken home, participants were instructed not to discuss the test with others until after they had completed all questions.

The interviewer and the test administrator filled in a behaviour rating form (Appendix 6) describing observations on the behaviour during the follow-up. In addition, the interviewer prepared a 'vignette' of each subject which described in narrative form pertinent observations in an attempt to characterize the person as well as possible, and stressing information which would not normally be documented by formal testing or rating scales.

## 5. Strategy of Analysis

All interview and test forms were marked with an identification number rather than a name. All data were transcribed and coded for computer processing. Records of additional findings, comments or observations not suitable for quantitative analysis were kept for further analysis.

The data analysis proceeded in the following steps:

a) Summary statistics (means, standard deviations, kurtosis, etc.) were calculated for the four groups and submitted to a four-group analysis of variance for continuous variables and to chi-square analysis for noncontinuous variables.

Using a large number of statistical tests such as the analyses of variance or the chi-square analysis as required for the many pieces of information and tests in this comprehensive follow-up study raises the risk of type 1 errors, i.e., at a $p$ level of $< .05$ for the rejection of the null-hypothesis, it must be expected that approximately 5 out of 100 analyses may produce significant results by chance alone. In order to reduce the danger of accepting differences (i.e., rejecting the null hypothesis) when they in fact may have been incurred by chance, a basic rule was followed: if in any set of similar variables analyzed, the majority of analyses tended to be significant, the danger of a type 1 error was considered minimal; when in a set of analyses only one or two significant findings occurred, these were considered suspect, and conclusions from them were appropriately qualified (see also under item [i] below).

b) Groups of related variables from a specific area (i.e., relating to health adjustment; neurological variables; employment etc.) were submitted to factor analysis, followed by discriminant function analysis between the four groups to explore group differences in multivariate fashion. This procedure, as well as the inclusion of Phase I data (thus making this a three-occasion analysis), tends to reduce or even eliminate the regression towards the mean effect; in fact, egression from the mean is equally likely to occur in more than single-variable 2-occasion designs than regression (Nesselroade, Stigler & Baltes 1980).

c) A correlational analysis of all repeated measures, i.e., the neurological and test data given at the time of the initial referral and at the Phase II follow-up across groups and within each group was conducted to study long-term changes with age. These results also can be viewed as a measure of stability (reliability) over time.

18

d) A breakdown of the LD groups into general and specific LD groups was attempted on the basis of achievement test and school grade data. These newly established groups were then contrasted in a manner similar to analyses a) and b) above with covariance analysis for age, sex, and intelligence as necessary, for the full range of outcome variables. This analysis was aimed at the usefulness of the currently used subgroupings ('types') of LD in terms of long-term outcome.

e) A separate analysis addressed the problem of subgrouping of LD empirically (Section 21). Subgroups of LD were formed on the basis of test results (including achievement tests) at the time of referral using hierarchical grouping analysis. Subgroups were also searched for on the basis of test results at Phase II testing. The obtained groups were then compared in order to see how such subgrouping changes over the follow-up period of 15 years (Spreen & Haaf 1986).

f) A number of predictor variables obtained at the time of the original referral were considered in relation to all major outcome variables at follow-up I and II. This analysis, presented by Spreen and Lawriw (1980), was repeated including Phase II long-term outcome variables and neuro-psychological repeat examination data.

g) A number of intervention and treatment variables obtained during follow-up I and II were considered in relation to long-term outcome (Section 26). An attempt was made to form several intervention and treatment groups, to eliminate major covariances, and to examine treatment effects by means of discriminant function analysis (e.g., treated vs. untreated).

h) Since intelligence may be an important factor in the outcome in many different areas, its effects were analyzed by a specific breakdown into intelligence level subgroups or by covariance as appropriate. In addition, the four groups were equated (force-matched) for IQ by eliminating some subjects, and repeating analyses with the four groups balanced for IQ (Section 24).

i) The effect of parents' socio-economic status on outcome was explored by canonical analysis (Section 20).

j) The generalizability of our results to other populations remains a problem, even though our sample appears to be reasonably representative of West Coast Canadian populations. Estimates of the true range of variability even within our subject population are possible, however, by various statistical manipulations. For example, one may use jack-knife procedures in the analysis of multi-variable sets, and to make a large number of different random split-half cross-validation tests or to apply the somewhat more sophisticated, but similar 'bootstrap' procedure (Diaconis & Efron 1983, Lunneborg 1985), as appropriate. The latter technique is also appropriate for data which violate the assumption of bivariate normality of distribution.

19

# B. RESULTS AND DISCUSSION
## a. Descriptive Data and Group Comparison

### 6. Living Arrangements and Parent and Sibling Relationships

Several questions relating to the living arrangements of our participants and to their parents and siblings were asked both at the Phase I (age 18) and Phase II (age 25) interview. Relationships with parents and friends have been reported as a significant factor in the development and the adult outcome of at risk and normal populations. For example, Jessor and Jessor (1984) found both parental support and parent-friend compatibility as significant contributors to the avoidance of 'deviant' behaviour and marijuana use. Herbst and Roesler (1986) considered social background and integration in considerable detail, and found that inappropriate or poor home environment (single parent family, unskilled mother, socio-economic status of parents) was present in 40.68% of their participants. They formed a 'social risk index' which was related to a variety of outcome variables.

At age 18, 67% of our participants still lived at home. However, there was a significant difference between groups: more subjects of Group 1 and of Group 4 (controls) lived at home (Table 6-1). For the control group subjects, this is probably a reflection of the fact that many of them were still attending school or college. At time II, this had changed significantly: while almost 53% of our brain-damaged group still lived at home, only between 26 and 30% of the other groups did. Forty-five percent of those

*Table 6-1: Living Arrangements at Phase I and II*

| Group | 1 | 2 | 3 | Control |
|---|---|---|---|---|
| Phase I | | | | |
| Living with parents | 78.5 | 53.5 | 63.6 | 74.5 |

chi-square = 11.21, $p < .01$

| | | | | |
|---|---|---|---|---|
| Phase II | | | | |
| Living with parents | 52.7 | 30.5 | 26.9 | 29.4 |
| Living alone | 14.5 | 28.8 | 23.1 | 7.8 |
| Sharing | 32.7 | 40.7 | 50.0 | 62.7 |

chi-square = 10.02, $p < .004$

21

of those sharing:

| with | | | | |
|---|---|---|---|---|
| wife/husband | 52.6 | 45.8 | 66.7 | 81.3 |
| sibling | 0 | 4.2 | 0 | 6.3 |
| friend | 5.3 | 25.0 | 16.7 | 9.4 |
| residence, group home | 42.1 | 25.0 | 16.7 | 3.1 |

chi-square $= 18.48, p < .03$

who had left home were sharing accommodations with somebody else, most often in the control group. Most of them shared with a husband or wife (81%), a reflection also of the larger percentage of married subjects in the control group.

An analysis of the age when subjects had left their parents' home showed a significant difference (Table 6-2). Subjects in Groups 2 and 3 left home more than a year earlier (at age 18) than subjects in Groups 1 and 4.

*Table 6-2: Age when Subjects First Left Home*

| Group 1 | Group 2 | Group 3 | Control |
|---|---|---|---|
| 19.88 | 18.42 | 18.25 | 19.84 |

$F=3.465 \, p < .02$

A significant difference between groups emerged at age 18 when subjects were asked whether they had 'lost' a parent for any reason (died, divorced, moved to another foster home etc.).This happened most frequently for subjects in group 1. During the Phase II interview this result was confirmed: subjects in Group 1 had, on average, 'lost' a parent more often than subjects in the other two LD groups. The smallest number of parents 'lost' was reported by the control group. Table 6-3 shows the number of subjects

*Table 6-3: Divorce and Change in Parents*

| Group<br>Type of Change | 1 | 2 | 3 | Control |
|---|---|---|---|---|
| Divorce, Phase I | 30.8 | 14.1 | 11.8 | 11.8 |
| | chi-square $= 10.11, p < .01$ | | | |
| Divorce, Phase II | 20.0 | 7.4 | 4.0 | 8.3 |
| | chi-square $= 6.58, p < .08$ | | | |
| Lost a parent for any other reason, Phase I | 21.0 | 7.2 | 2.9 | 7.8 |
| Phase II | 38.8 | 19.2 | 25.7 | 11.8. |
| | chi-square $= 31.8, p < .006$ | | | |

22

in each group who reported a divorce of parents during the period preceding the Phase I interview or between the Phase I and Phase II interview. The divorce rate for Group 1 is particularly striking (30%) while the other three groups had divorce rates between 14 and 11%. Asked how many 'fathers' the participants had, a significantly higher number for subjects in group 1 was found, and the number reported by group 4 was lower than for all other groups (means: 1.21, 1.10, 1.12, 1.02, $F[3] = 2.15$, $p < .09$). Since this difference was not significant for 'mothers', this suggests that the participants usually stayed with the mother after divorce.

The median number of other people living with our participants was four (means: 4.71, 4.38, 3.88, 4.56, chi square = 60.22, $p < .001$).

Much attention has been paid to the question whether firstborn or later born children are more frequent among LD children. Our analysis found no significant differences in birthrank, nor were there more twins among our participants in any of the groups.

No significant differences between groups were found for the question whether both parents were still alive. Of our subjects, 8.6% reported that they had been physically abused as a child, but no significant group differences were found.

In *summary*, a greater proportion of our LD groups with minimal or no neurological impairment left home earlier and lived on their own more often. The control group stayed with parents (and in school) more frequently, but at age 25 a majority lived with husband or wife. The LD group with definite neurological impairment also stayed at home longer, but at age 25 many of them lived in group home or shared/apartment situations. The divorce rate of parents for this group is strikingly high and may be a reflection of the stress on the family with neurologically impaired children. No support for the effect of birthrank or for an increased amount of child abuse in LD children could be found.

### 7.Education

The educational career of our participants was examined in detail in collaboration with Denbigh (1979), and included the permanent school record data. During Phase II, several questions of the Phase I study were reanalyzed together with additional questions posed during the interview.

Seventy-eight percent of our subjects entered preschool at a mean age of 4.5 years. There was no difference between groups on these means, although some subjects in group 1 entered preschool earlier than those in the other groups. Preschool attendence lasted an average of 11.4 months (no difference between groups). School entry was at age 5.8, for all groups. At the time of the Phase I interview, 41% of our subject still attended school

Table 7-1: Highest School Grade Completed by Group (in %)

| Group | 1 | 2 | 3 | Control |
|---|---|---|---|---|
| *Highest Grade Completed* | | | | |
| < 10 | 26.1 | 20.4 | 23.0 | 0 |
| 10 | 25.9 | 33.9 | 34.6 | 2.0 |
| 11 | 7.4 | 8.5 | 7.7 | 0 |
| 12 | 40.7 | 37.3 | 34.6 | 98.0 |

chi-square $= 68.21, p < .001$

(69% of the control group, 39, 33 and 31% of groups 1-3). At the Phase II interview , the three LD groups had completed significantly fewer grades than the control group ($p < .001$). Among the LD groups, group 3 had the lowest grade 12 completion level (Table 7-1). Programs completed were more often 'academic' for the control group and 'general' (occupational) for the LD groups (Table 7-2). Ninety-eight percent of the control group left school after completion of the last grade attended, while only 63, 65, and 61% of groups 1-3 completed their last grade. Their school attendence, therefore, had not only been shortened, but also seriously disrupted.

*Table 7-2: Type of School Program Attended (in %)*

| Group | 1 | 2 | 3 | Control |
|---|---|---|---|---|
| *Program* | | | | |
| academic | 26.5 | 30.5 | 38.5 | 84.3 |
| modified | 6.1 | 3.4 | 3.8 | 2.0 |
| general | 67.3 | 66.1 | 57.7 | 13.7 |

chi-square $= 44.59, p < .001$

For comparison, the following data provided by the Greater Victoria School Board for the year 1977/78 (comparable to the later school years of our subjects) may be of interest. During that year, a total of 636 children in grades 7 to 11, or 6% of the total school population of 11,655 pupils, left school (primary reasons given: to seek employment, poor attendance, underachievement, etc.). Specifically, in grade 7, 52 or 3% of the school population, in grade 8, 84 or 4%, in grade 9, 171 or 9%, in grade 10, 206 or 11%, in grade 11, 123 or 5.6% of the total population in the respective grades left during that year. As can be seen from Table 7-1, school leaving occurred considerably more frequently in our population compared to the general population of the school district.

There was a significant difference between groups in the number of subjects who said they needed special help in school: Only 43% of the control subjects answered this question with yes while 87, 88, and 89% of group 1 to 3 subjects answered in the affirmative.

Asked whether they did receive special help in school (special class, special instruction, tutoring), 38% of the control group said yes; the corresponding figures for groups 1 to 3 were 92, 84, and 84%. Private tutoring or instruction were received as early as grade 1 by 40% of the participants. However, this instruction was remedial for 24, 54, and 43% of groups 1 to 3, while our control group received such help later (during grade 2) and was advanced rather than remedial. Only about 16% of our subjects attended summer school, usually in grade 6, 7, or 8. Again, for groups 1 to 3, summer school was mainly to help them catch up with their curriculum, while for more than a third of the control group summer school provided advanced instruction. All three LD groups received more help from family members than group 4.

Thirty-two percent of the subjects in group 3 disliked school, while subjects in groups 1 and 2 said they 'did not like it very much' or 'it's ok', and the majority of subjects in the control group said 'it's ok' or that they really loved it ($p < .01$). This difference in attitude towards school was still present during the Phase II interview, although the differences were slightly less pronounced ($p < .028$). No significant shifts in attitude from the first to the second interview occurred.

A negative attitudinal shift during the last four years of school towards academic achievement and a positive shift towards independence has been reported in longitudinal studies of high-school samples (Jessor & Jessor 1984). This is reflected in our sample by a significantly lower involvement in extracurricular activities at school and in significant group differences. On a 1 to 4 scale (from no involvement to strong involvement) the group means were 2.3, 2.4, 2.6, and 3.0 respectively. Our participants reported that they spent 1.4, 2.7, 3.2, and 3.8 hours per week on such activities.

A significantly higher number of subjects in group 3 (36.4%), but also a larger number of subjects in groups 1 (18.5%) and 2 (18.6%) were expelled or suspended from school at least once (Controls 3.9%, $p < .006$). Significantly more males (22.5%) than females (3.5%) were expelled, while on all other school questions sex differences were not significant.

A significantly higher proportion of group 4 (control) subjects (47.1%) took college or university academic courses than group 1, 2, or 3 subjects (15, 12, and 12% respectively).

While over 90% of control subjects had never spent any time in special classes of any kind, 64.6% of group 1, 57.6% of group 2, and 46.2% of group 3 had been in such classes as explored in the Phase I interview, many of them for several grades. However, the number of times they received special instruction or the number of grades in which they had a learning-assistance teacher was relatively small and did not differ significantly between groups. Special assistance was remedial for 83.8, 86.4, and 76.9%

25

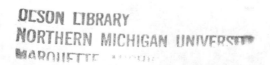

of groups 1 to 3 respectively, but only for 49% of group 4. On the other hand, 11.8% of our group 4 subjects had received special assistance for advanced training while virtually none of the group 1 to 3 subjects had such assistance.

The LD samples were restricted to those with IQs of 90 or more ($n = 21$, 37, and 19 respectively) to calculate grade point averages (GPA) from the schools' permanent record card. GPAs are calculated on a scale of 1 to 7 with 1 indicating failure and 7 representing a grade of A. The GPA in academic subjects (language arts, arithmetic, social studies), for elective school subjects and for physical education are shown in Table 7-3.

*Table 7-3: Grade Point Averages in School for Participants with an IQ > 90*

| Group | Academic Subjects | Art | Music | Home Educ. | Indust-rial Ed. | Commerce | Physical Educ. |
|---|---|---|---|---|---|---|---|
| BD | 3.5 | 4.3 | 5.1 | 4.1 | 4.1 | 3.6 | 4.5 |
| MBD | 3.8 | 4.6 | 5.1 | 4.5 | 4.2 | 4.0 | 4.4 |
| LD | 4.0 | 4.8 | 5.1 | 4.5 | 4.8 | 3.4 | 4.6 |
| Controls | 4.9 | 5.1 | 5.1 | 5.4 | 5.0 | 5.1 | 4.7 |

The difference between LD subjects and controls in academic subjects as well as in art, home economics, industrial education and commerce were significant at the .01 level, while the difference in music and physical education was not. The average highest grade level completed by this restricted sample was 10.8, 10.7, 11.1, and 11.6 respectively for the four groups at age 19 ($F[3, 120] = 18.8$; $p < .001$ comparing the three LD with the control group).

In all schools attended by our participants it was common practice to present awards, honours, or prizes. Our groups differed from control subjects in two ways: the LD subjects usually received the more common, nonacademic awards ('citizenship award'); more rare awards were only occasionally reported in group 2 and 3 subjects, but more frequently in the control group as many as 5 awards, while only 22, 24, and 11 subjects of groups 3, 2, and 1 received that many awards.

LD subjects were also less frequently nominated or elected as officer of a school class, club, or other organization than controls (24, 27, 31, and 62% respectively for groups 1 to 4).

During the second interview (Phase II) a significantly higher number of LD subjects remembered special problems in mathematics (46% in group 1, 52 and 66% in groups 2 and 3, 26% in the control group). When asked during the Phase II interview whether they still experienced problems in mathematics, 82.3, 93.1, and 88% of groups 1 to 3 answered in the affirmative and a large proportion (21.6, 31, and 32%) described these problems as severe, while only 38.5% of the control group had 'slight' and

26

11.5% still had 'moderate' problems. There was a significant linear decrease from group 1 to 4 in the number of subjects who said that these problems had affected their choice of jobs, schools etc. (52.0, 45.6, 26.9, 16.0%, $p<.009$, no significant sex difference). The types of school problems are detailed in Table 7-4. Problems in reading and spelling were most frequent.

*Table 7-4: Reported Problems in Reading, Spelling, Speaking or Writing Affecting School Progress - Phase II Interview*

| Group | 1 | 2 | 3 | 4 (in %) |
|---|---|---|---|---|
| Problem | | | | |
| none | 21.8 | 22.0 | 34.6 | 84.3 |
| reading | 27.3 | 5.1 | 7.7 | 3.9 |
| spelling | 10.9 | 15.3 | 26.9 | 7.8 |
| speaking | 3.6 | 1.7 | 0 | 0 |
| writing | 0 | 1.7 | 0 | 0 |
| written expression | 1.8 | 0 | 0 | 0 |
| reading and spelling | 25.5 | 33.9 | 26.9 | 2.0 |
| multiple problems | 9.1 | 20.4 | 3.8 | 2.0 |

chi-square $= 89.89$, $p < .001$

There was a significant difference between groups on the question whether either of their natural parents had problems in reading. The total percentage of participants reporting such problems in their parents ranged from 23 to 32 with the highest numbers found in group 3. Slightly more females than males reported such parental disabilities ($p < .07$). In contrast, parental problems in mathematics were reported very infrequently and no group differences were found.

There was no group difference in the number of subjects who still attended school during the 5 years preceding the Phase II interview, and those who did, did not differ significantly by group in the reported grades received. This seems to indicate that for most of our clients education is essentially completed so that the results on employment and income are less likely to be affected by the fact that a portion of the subjects still attend school. Subjects in the control group who did attend any school, evening course etc. were more likely attending university, while the former LD subjects reported more vocational training and high school completion programs.

A special analysis was carried out for subjects who said that they had received no special help in school. As Table 7-5 shows, between 11 and 50% of these subjects reported that they did experience problems, mainly in the language/reading/spelling areas. As expected, a significant group difference was found for this question. A similar group difference existed for those subjects who did receive special help in school.

*Table 7-5: Problems in School Reported by Participants Who Did not Receive Special Help in School - Phase II Interview*

| Group | 1 | 2 | 3 | Control |
|---|---|---|---|---|
| *Problem* | | | | |
| none | 71.4 | 50.0 | 33.3 | 89.7 |
| reading | 14.3 | 16.7 | 0 | 6.9 |
| spelling | 0 | 0 | 66.7 | 3.4 |
| reading, spelling and/or speaking | 14.3 | 33.4 | 0 | 0 |
| mathematics | 42.9 | 33.3 | 66.7 | 6.9 |

chi-square for non-mathematics problems = 15.65, $p < .010$
chi-square for mathematics problems = 10.15, $p < .017$

Part of the results on the education of our participants were reanalyzed with the three LD groups equated for IQ at the time of referral. Eliminating the IQ differences did not change the results. In fact, the results for 'need special help in school', taking academic courses at college or university, 'how did you like school', and for expulsion from school were even more pronounced and significant (for suspension and expulsion: 22, 18, 34.5, and 3.5% for groups 1 to 4 respectively).

One additional result emerged from this reanalysis: while most subjects had attended preschool an average of 10 months, more subjects in group 1 and 2 attended longer ( up to 20 and 30 months; $p < .09$). This is probably a reflection of the fact that more of our subjects in these groups were held back for a year or even 2 years before entering grade 1.

In *summary*, a significantly higher proportion of all three LD groups left school from a lower grade than the control group or the general school population of the district. They often left school in the middle rather than at the end of the school year, stated that they needed and received special help at school more often, attended a general rather than an academic program, were more often expelled or suspended from school, and reported a more negative attitude towards school. Only 1 or 2 out of 10 took college or university courses as compared to 4 or 5 in controls. In school, they received lower grades and fewer awards. The proportion of parents with reading problems was significantly higher in our LD population, especially in the group of LD without neurological findings.

## 8. Employment

Employment and vocational achievement during the adult years rank among the most serious concerns for LD populations. Previous studies have shown contradictory results and are mostly based on relatively early follow-up (age 18 or 19) when a substantial part of the population is still attending school or post-high-school education programs.

Early studies by Balow and Blomquist (1965), Preston and Yarington (1967), Rawson (1968), and Robinson and Smith (1972) all reported vocational outcomes comparable to their age-peers, and Rawson even found that her dyslexic population, enrolled in private extensive remediation programs, completed college and showed no difference in occupational achievement compared to normal reading control subjects. A recent study by Bruck (1985) seems to confirm these findings. Gottfredson, Finucci, and Childs (1983), in a follow-up of alumni of a private secondary school at adult age, found that these alumni were more successful in occupational achievement than the alumni of a control school in spite of the reading handicap, because of the high socio-economic status of their families. Compared to their fathers, however, mildly dyslexic alumni were found more often in management and sales jobs, and less often in professional jobs because they less often obtained Bachelors or advanced degrees than their fathers. Severely dyslexic alumni were found more often in blue-collar jobs than mildly disabled men. The authors attribute these findings to the need for reading, writing, and educational credentials in professional jobs while in managerial and sales jobs initiative, responsibility, persuasiveness, and competitiveness are primary requirements.

Unfortunately, these studies tended to use highly restrictive samples (upper socio-economic class, high mean IQ) matched for total years of education and failed to provide a region-specific representative control group. This restricts the possibility to generalize from these findings. Other authors (e.g., Washburn 1975) reported that 75% of LD secondary-school students leave school unemployed and without plans for a job or job training. Katz-Garris et al. (1983) reported that in a vocational rehabilitation center only 48.5% of LD subjects had 'successful case closure' compared to a 70.5% success rate in all disabilities groups. Blalock (1982) documented frequent job changes and misunderstandings with employers for adult LD clients. Herbst and Roesler (1986) found that occupation and frequency of job changes was directly related to IQ in their group. Only 41% had obtained a driver's licence and 33% were exempted as unfit from military service (compulsary in East Germany).

The contradictory findings of different studies are most likely due to differences in sampling. The relatively broad and fairly large sample of the current study may provide some clarification.

During the Phase I interview, 72% of our subjects were working; between 35 and 41% of the three LD groups and 60% of our controls were still in school, a reflection of the early school leaving of LD subjects and the continuing education of control subjects.

Most subjects had had some part-time job during their school years such as paper-route, delivery, babysitting, day care, etc. A significant difference between groups was found for the age when they first started these jobs:

29

group 1 started at an average age of 15.5, group 2 at age 14.4, group 3 at age 14.1, and the control group at age 13.2. Nearly all (97%) of our subjects had done jobs around the home or for friends and neighbors, but significantly more subjects in group 1 reported liking such jobs; a linear trend emerged across the four groups with group 4 (controls) liking such jobs 'sometimes, only rarely'.

The main source of income at Phase I was not significantly different between groups, but a trend towards more social-assistance and unemployment income in groups 1 and 2, and more reliance on income from jobs was evident for groups 3 and 4 (Table 8-1). At the Phase II interview the difference between groups in source of income was highly significant (Table 8-2).

*Table 8-1: Main Source of Income\* at Phase I*

| Group | 1 | 2 | 3 | 4 |
|-------|---|---|---|---|
| *Source* | | | | |
| Parents only | 42.2 | 28.2 | 29.0 | 45.1 |
| Welfare/Social Assistance | 10.9 | 8.5 | 3.2 | 0 |
| Unemployment Insurance | 1.6 | 4.2 | 0 | 0 |
| Job | 18.8 | 39.4 | 41.9 | 33.3 |
| Other | 26.6 | 19.7 | 25.8 | 21.6 |

* includes multiple sources of income

*Table 8-2: Sources of Income\* at Phase II*

| Group | 1 | 2 | 3 | 4 |
|-------|---|---|---|---|
| *Source* | | | | |
| Parent's Income | 16.4 | 5.1 | 7.7 | 3.9 |
| Social Assistance | 27.3 | 11.9 | 11.5 | 0 |
| Unemployment Insurance | 5.5 | 5.1 | 11.5 | 2.0 |
| Own Job | 41.8 | 64.4 | 53.8 | 88.2 |
| Spouse's Income | 3.6 | 8.5 | 11.5 | 3.9 |
| Other | 5.5 | 5.1 | 3.8 | 2.0 |

chi-square $= 37.5, p < .001$.
* includes multiple sources of income.

Including part-time or temporary or sheltered employment, 69.3% of our subjects were employed at the time of the Phase I interview. This figure had risen only slightly (70.7%) at the time of the Phase II interview (Table 8-3). The table shows a highly significant group difference at both times: 88.2% of the control group were employed compared to 60, 73, and 54% in groups 1, 2, and 3 respectively. The employment figure for the control

*Table 8-3: Percentage of Participants Employed*
*at Phase I and Phase II Interview*

| Group | 1 | 2 | 3 | 4 |
|---|---|---|---|---|
| *Employed* | | | | |
| Phase I | 58.6 | 66.7 | 80.0 | 78.4 |
| Phase II | 60.0 | 72.9 | 53.8 | 88.2 |

chi-square $= 14.31, p < .002$

*Table 8-4: Percentage of Participants Having*
*Difficulty Finding a Job, Phase I and Phase II*

| Group | 1 | 2 | 3 | 4 |
|---|---|---|---|---|
| Phase I | 54.5 | 19.6 | 16.0 | 4.2 |
| Phase II | 55.1 | 36.5 | 26.9 | 7.8 |

chi-square $= 26.49, p < .001$

group is close to the employment rate in British Columbia at the time of the interview recorded by Statistics Canada (Canada Employment and Immigration, Victoria, B.C.) for the 20- to 24-year age group in January of 1982 (a date close to the time of the actual interviews). For the 15- to 19-year age group the unemployment rate in the Western B.C. area was 20.7%. For the 20- to 24-year old group the unemployment rate was 13.9% and for the general population of B.C. 9.8%. These figures rose in August 1982 to 24.3, 20.5, and 13.1 respectively (part of this rise is due to the inclusion of high-school and university students seeking employment during the summer months). The Statistics Canada figures are based on a procedure similar to our own survey, namely on a phone survey of households, inquiring about the number of people currently employed or seeking employment.

Compared to the Phase I interview, the employment rate of the two brain-dysfunction groups remained stable while employment for the LD group without neurological impairment dropped from 80 to 54%. Table 8-4 indicates that our participants had experienced difficulty in finding a job with increasing degree as neurological impairment increased, i.e., 7.8% of the control subjects reported difficulties, whereas 51% of Group 1 (definite neurological impairment) experienced difficulties in finding employment, a significant linear trend at both interviews. Changes in jobs (reflected in the number of jobs held during the last five years, Table 8-5) showed no significant group differences.

*Table 8-5: Number of Jobs Held During 5 Years
Preceding Phase II Interview*

| Group | 1 | 2 | 3 | 4 |
|---|---|---|---|---|
| *Number of Jobs* | | | | |
| 0 | 7.3 | 5.1 | 3.8 | 0 |
| 1 | 21.8 | 25.4 | 15.4 | 25.5 |
| 2 | 14.5 | 18.6 | 11.5 | 19.6 |
| 3 | 16.4 | 23.7 | 11.5 | 15.7 |
| 4 or more | 40.0 | 27.1 | 57.7 | 39.2 |

chi-square $= 11.91, p < .45$

A significant difference between groups was found for the type of jobs held (Table 8-6). The control group held skilled and advanced training jobs. Asked what type of job they would really like to obtain, the LD groups showed a less ambitious selection. A number of the group 1 subjects appeared to be expecting no more than their present type of employment.

*Table 8-6: Type of Job Held at Phase II Interview*

| Group | 1 | 2 | 3 | 4 |
|---|---|---|---|---|
| paper route | 0 | 1.8 | 0 | 0 |
| other deliveries | 7.8 | 3.6 | 4.0 | 3.9 |
| clerical | 3.9 | 0 | 0 | 5.9 |
| day care | 2.0 | 1.8 | 0 | 0 |
| sales, commission | 0 | 0 | 0 | 3.9 |
| sales | 2.0 | 1.8 | 0 | 9.8 |
| unskilled labor | 58.8 | 55.4 | 48.0 | 25.5 |
| skilled labor | 11.8 | 25.0 | 28.0 | 17.6 |
| own business | 2.0 | 1.8 | 8.0 | 3.0 |
| professional services | 0 | 0 | 0 | 13.7 |
| other | 11.8 | 8.9 | 12.0 | 15.7 |

chi square $= 53.58, p < .005$

A linear difference between groups which showed more temporary employment in Group 1 and more permanent employment in Group 4 approached significance (Table 8-7). This trend had not been evident at the Phase I interview, probably because a larger number of control group subjects were still in some form of education or training program.

The highest income during the last 5 years and the average income during the last five years both showed significant differences between groups. Al-though Group 3 surpassed the control group in highest income per month (probably due to seasonal employment, primarily logging), the average income showed a linear trend from group 1 ($887/month) to

*Table 8-7: Employment and Income at Phase II Interview*

| Group | 1 | 2 | 3 | 4 | $p<$ |
|---|---|---|---|---|---|
| Percent with permanent employment | 52.9 | 67.9 | 68.0 | 76.5 | .089 |
| monthly salary for longest held job | 887 | 1394 | 1381 | 1478 | .008 |
| highest monthly salary | 1124 | 1584 | 1824 | 1698 | .007 |

Group 4 ($1,478/month). A significant sex difference (females $1,058, males $1,374/month) was also evident. The difference between groups can be expected to become more pronounced in future years since control subjects were often still in the beginning stages of their career after extended schooling while many of the LD subjects had started their career earlier with fewer options in job choice (this in turn would tend to limit their salary increases over time).

In *summary*, we observed a linear trend on employment variables ranging from poorest outcome to best across the three LD groups to the control group. LD participants started part-time jobs later in their life, lived more often on social assistance or unemployment income, and showed a high unemployment rate compared to both the control group and the Statistics Canada figures for that time period. They had considerably more difficulty in finding a job, changed jobs more often, and were more often employed as unskilled laborers. Their monthly salary at the age of 25 was significantly lower even though many subjects in the control group delayed their entry into the labor market by extended schooling.

## 9. Health, Medication, and Drug Use

During the Phase II examination all participants were weighed and measured. The average height for males was 176.25 cm, for females 162.31 cm. No significant differences in height between the four groups were found, although group 1 and 2 females were slightly shorter on average (160.5 and 160.7 cm respectively). The average weight for males was 74.99 kg and for females 61.02 kg. Again, no significant group differences were found, although females in group 3 were somewhat heavier (67.1 kg) on average. In order to check whether a significantly larger number of overweight subjects were present in any of the groups, weights were recoded in terms of deviation from standard weights for males and females of this age group (Bray 1976). Two males and 9 females were underweight and 17 males and 28 females overweight, but no significant group differences were found.

During the Phase II interview and testing, the examiners rated each participant's stature as slender (markedly underweight), more slender than average, average, plump, and obese. The three LD groups received a significantly higher (median= average to plump) rating than the control group, and females were rated more towards the 'heavy' side than controls.

Pure tone hearing level was measured for all subjects for each ear at 500, 1000, 2000, and 4000 Hz. The 1000, 2000, and 4000 Hz thresholds were significantly elevated for males, particularly in group 2 (in mean dB) for both ears. With IQ-matched groups this difference was still significant for the high frequency range (Mean dB level 10.4, 11.2, 8.4, and 2.6 at 4000 Hz respectively). While the average dB levels are still within the 'normal' hearing range, a mild high frequency loss for these groups is noted.

The results were scanned for subjects who had a dB level of 20 and higher. This level, which approaches a significant hearing loss, was found in 34.3% of group 1 subjects, in 27.4% of group 2, and in 28.6% of group 3 subjects, while only 2 subjects (3.9%) in group 4 showed impairment at that level. The difference was significant, although significance dropped to .09 when groups were matched for IQ. More males than females showed such impairment.

Health Problems

During the Phase I interview with clients and parents a history of illnesses during infancy and childhood was obtained and coded (Hern 1979). A similar update interview was conducted during the Phase II interview.

In general, at Phase I health was more often impaired in females than in males, which may also account in part for the increased social difficulties in females. In addition, the number of central nervous system disorders, seizures, and problems of the mother during pregnancy and birth, decreased significantly from group 1 to group 4 (Table 9-1), i.e., with decreasing level of neurological impairment. General health and number of accidents were not significantly different between groups. For the Phase II reporting period, again no significant differences between groups in the number of accidents was found (59.3, 61.0, 61.5, and 52.9% of subjects had been involved in accidents of any kind during the reporting period). The total number of accidents for both reporting periods was also not significantly different between groups (no accidents for 10.4, 12.3, 17.1, and 13.7% respectively). This finding is contrary to previous research (Kinsbourne 1973; Wender 1971) which claimed that such children are 'accident prone'.

At the Phase II interview groups were also significantly different in reporting of seizure activity (18.2, 11.9, 4.0, and 0%). It appears that seizure activity did not change appreciably during the developmental period of our subjects up to young adulthood.

34

*Table 9-1: Health Problems During Childhood and Adolescence*

| Problem | BD | MBD | LD | C | $p<$* |
|---|---|---|---|---|---|
| n | 52 | 66 | 34 | 52 | |
| CNS Problems | 30 | 15 | 5 | 0 | .001 |
| Pregnancy & Birth | 26 | 26 | 10 | 8 | .001 |
| premature | 10 | 6 | 1 | 2 | |
| instrument delivery | 3 | 4 | 5 | 3 | |
| anoxia | 4 | 6 | 0 | 0 | |
| prolonged labour | 4 | 6 | 2 | 1 | |
| mother sick | 2 | 0 | 1 | 0 | |
| postmature | 1 | 2 | 0 | 1 | |
| caesarian | 1 | 2 | 1 | 0 | |
| ABO incompatibility | 1 | 0 | 0 | 1 | |
| Other Health Problems | 62 | 114 | 68 | 109 | .01 |
| Seizures | 23 | 14 | 4 | 3 | .001 |
| before referral | 23 | 14 | 3 | 0 | |
| between 10-18 years | 23 | 11 | 2 | 0 | |
| petit mal | 2 | 3 | 1 | 0 | |
| psychomotor | 3 | 2 | 0 | 0 | |
| Jacksonian | 6 | 2 | 1 | 0 | |
| grand mal | 10 | 7 | 2 | 1 | |
| febrile | 2 | 0 | 0 | 2 | |
| duration of seizure | | | | | |
| problem in months | 80 | 57 | 36 | <1 | |
| Abnormal EEG | | | | | |
| nonspecific | 17 | 29 | 0 | 0 | |
| right | 11 | 6 | 0 | 0 | |
| left | 14 | 6 | 0 | 0 | |
| dysrhythmia gr.2 | 6 | 20 | 0 | 0 | |
| dysrhythmia gr.3 | 29 | 3 | 0 | 0 | |
| delta gr.1 | 5 | 14 | 0 | 0 | |
| delta gr.2 | 6 | 3 | 0 | 0 | |
| delta gr.3 | 1 | 0 | 0 | 0 | |
| Frequency of Accidents | 31 | 36 | 28 | 25 | ns |

* chi-square using expected frequencies for each group.

Suicide attempts were reported by very few subjects and no significant group differences were found (3.6, 8.5, 7.7, and 0%, 7% female, 3.7% male).

Subjects were asked whether their health problems prevented or limited their ability to drive a motor vehicle. Thirteen percent of group 1, 6.8% of group 2, 3.8% of group 3, and 0% of group 4 answered in the affirmative.

## Drugs and Medication

A series of questions explored the use of prescription medication, over-the-counter and street drugs. During the Phase I interview, significantly more subjects in group 1 had used medication, and the total number of medications used was also higher. Little information could be obtained in terms of drug effectiveness, and no difference between groups was found when asked whether they were currently on medication (55 to 67% said yes). Groups 1 and 2 took medication for significantly longer periods (165 and 134 months) than groups 3 and 4 (95 and 43 months). The purpose of prescriptions ranged from brief medications for minor infections to lengthy ones for seizures and hyperactivity.

During the second interview, tranquilizer use was between 11 and 19% in groups 1 to 3 and 5.9% in group 4. No group differences were found in the use of antibiotics. Antipsychotic drugs were only used by 3 subjects in group 1 and 1 subject in group 2, antidepressants by 1 subject in group 1 and 2 subjects in group 2. The use of anticonvulsants was significantly different between groups as expected: 20% in group 1, 6.8% in group 2, and 3.8% in group 3 but none in group 4. Only 3 subjects in group 1 used antiparkinsonian medication. The use of stimulant medication was admitted by only one subject in groups 1 and 4 each. Painkillers were used by 10.9% in group 1, 25.4% in group 2, 26.9% in group 3, and 13.7% in group 4 (n.s.); sedatives by between 5.9% (group 4) and 11.9% (group 2) of our subjects (n.s.); respiratory drugs by 6 subjects in group 4 only; and thyroid medication by a small number of subjects in groups 1, 2, and 4 (n.s.). No significant difference between groups was found for antiallergic medication or gastric and other types of medication, including headache remedies. However, the total drug use (total number of drugs taken) differed significantly between sexes with females taking more medication.

Forty percent of group 1, 35.8% of group 2, 57.1% of group 3, and 38.8% of group 4 reported during the Phase I interview that they had taken street drugs at least once (no significant group difference). There was also no significant group difference in alcohol use or the admission of having a problem in handling alcohol during adolescence as reported in the Phase I interview.

During the phase II interview use of street drugs (nonmedical) during the 5 years preceding the interview was admitted by 80% of group 1 subjects, 84.5% of group 2, 96.2% of group 3, and 92.2% of group 4 (n.s.). Males used marijuana more frequently, but no group differences existed for this, nor were differences found for LSD and cocaine. No subjects admitted the use of heroin or amphetamines. Males used street drugs significantly more than females. No group differences were found in the frequency of street drug use.

Frequency of alcohol use was significantly different between groups with the control group using alcohol most frequently and group 1 subjects least frequently. Males again used alcohol more frequently than females.

In *summary* our LD participants stature was more often rated as heavy or plump although weight and height differences were not significant as compared to controls. They had significantly higher hearing thresholds, in some subjects approaching mild hearing loss, and reported more health problems, both at birth and in childhood as well as seizures. The LD groups were more often seen by a psychiatrist or psychologist. Groups 1 and 2, especially females, received more prescription medication, and for longer periods, most often tranquilizers. Street drugs and alcohol were used by all groups, including controls, with similar frequency.

## 10. Social Adjustment

Similar to the occupational outcome, previous studies have shown a wide variety of results concerning the long-term social adjustment of former LD students (Connolly 1969; Helper 1980; Spreen 1982). The results range from good social adjustment to serious maladjustment, antisocial behaviour and poor relationships with family members, spouse, and friends. Herbst and Roesler (1986) reported that their follow-up participants at the mean age of 22 had fewer sexual relationships, and that 33% of their male subjects never had a sexual relationship at all.

Questions relating to the participants' relation to parents, siblings, and friends were asked at both the age 18 and the age 25 interview. The first set of questions referred to the relationship between and with the parents. No significant group differences were found on the question how their parents were getting along with each other, nor did our participants show a difference between the earlier and later reporting date. No significant difference was found between groups when asked how they were getting along with mother or father. However, more subjects in the control group and fewer subjects in Group 1 reported getting along 'very well' with their siblings at age 25 (Table 10-1). This difference had not been found at the Phase I interview and probably reflects a more mature adjustment to siblings in the control group and more tension in the LD and particularly in the brain-damaged groups.

*Table 10-1: Interviewee's Reported Ability to Get Along With Siblings*
*Phase II Interview*

| Group | 1 | 2 | 3 | Control |
|---|---|---|---|---|
| Getting Along | | | | |
| Poor | 3.8 | 1.7 | 8.3 | 0 |
| Satisfactory | 37.7 | 34.5 | 25.0 | 16.0 |
| Very Good | 58.5 | 63.8 | 66.7 | 84.0 |

chi-square $= 12.34, p < .05$

A significant difference between groups was found at the Phase I interview for the question whether they had ever 'dated' (Table 10-2). The difference was mainly between groups 1 and 2 as compared to groups 3 and 4. Dating was much more common among girls (86%) than boys (69%). The group difference was even more pronounced at the Phase II interview. Even at that relatively late age, over 40% of the Group 1 participants had never dated.

*Table 10-2: Percentage of Participants Who Had Dated at Phase I and Phase II Interview.*

| Group | 1 | 2 | 3 | Control |
|---|---|---|---|---|
| Phase I | 63.3 | 66.7 | 92.6 | 87.2 |
| Phase II | 59.5* | 73.2 | 90.9 | 100.0 |

chi-square $= 14.48, p < .002$

* slight change in percentages due to change of number of participants in Phase II.

There was no significant group difference between the number of close friends listed by our participants, although Group 1 subjects reported to have more casual rather than close friends compared to subjects in the other groups. Phone calls to friends were most frequent in the control group, less in group 3 than in group 2 and least in group 1, a significant difference between the control group and the LD groups.

Sex of friends at age 18 was not significantly different for the four groups, but girls tended to have more friends of the opposite sex than boys. Girls also reported that they had more casual friends to talk to them on the phone than boys. No significant differences between groups were found on the questions of how they get along with friends, whether they were satisfied with them, how many dates they had during the last 3 months, and how often they and their friends visited each other.

Behaviour problems during childhood and adolescence were reported for 41, 49, 32, and 21% of our subjects respectively ($p < .01$). Such problems were noted first around age 8 and lasted an average of 7 to 8 years (no significant difference between groups). In our question, behaviour problems were defined inclusively (e.g. problems of discipline, anxiety, depression, hyperactivity etc.). Behaviour problems persisted or occurred for the first time after the time of referral in 52, 52, 33, and 21% of the participants ($p < .001$). Asked whether they had a problem which parents and/or teachers did not recognize, 55, 50, 45, and 19% answered in the affirmative ($p < .001$).

## Hobbies and Recreation

Participants listed their hobbies during both interviews. The hobbies were coded according to their general nature and a count of each type of hobby was carried out. In general, participants in group 1 listed fewer hobbies, but a significant group difference was found for hobbies 'around the house' (watching TV, collecting, caring for pets, gardening, reading, housework). As shown in Table 10-3, this type of hobby was less frequent in group 3 as compared to other groups. Sixty-two percent of Group 1 subjects mentioned as many as four different house-related hobbies. In contrast, both sports-oriented hobbies and social activities were more frequent in group 1 (Table 10-4).

*Table 10-3: Percentage of Subjects Involved in*
*Hobbies Around the House at Phase I and II Follow-Up*

| Group | 1 | 2 | 3 | Control |
|---|---|---|---|---|
| Phase I | 82.1 | 86.3 | 77.1 | 96.1 |
| | Chi-square = 33.35, $p < .04$ | | | |
| Phase II | 67.2 | 52.1 | 45.7 | 74.5 |
| | chi-square = 19.76, $p < .02$ | | | |

*Table 10-4: Percentage of Subjects Involved in*
*Sports-Oriented and Social Activities at Phase I Follow-Up*

| Group | 1 | 2 | 3 | Control |
|---|---|---|---|---|
| Sports-Oriented | 62.7 | 67.1 | 77.1 | 90.2 |
| | Chi-square = 40.05, $p < .007$ | | | |
| Social Activ. | 68.7 | 53.4 | 51.4 | 94.1 |
| | chi-square = 49.31, $p < .001$ | | | |

Strikingly, 31, 47, and 49% of groups 1, 2, and 3 respectively had no social activities listed as hobbies while only 6% of the controls had no such hobby. Another difference between the control and the LD groups at Phase I was found for "organized group recreation", which was much higher for the control group (37.3 vs. 15.9%).

Amongst these differences obtained at the Phase I interview the difference for house-type hobbies remained significant at Phase II, while the differences for social and sports activities lost significance (mainly because of decreasing interest in the control group). Hobbies of the arts and 'motor and mechanics' variety did not differ significantly between groups in either interview.

In *summary*, the relationship with the family did not differ between groups at age 18, but at age 25 the control group reported a better relationship with siblings than the LD groups. Dating was less common in males than in females, and less frequent in the neurologically impaired groups. At age 25, as many as 40% of our group 1 subjects had never dated. Behaviour problems were more common in LD subjects. Controls reported more sports-oriented and social activities at age 18 while group 1 had more hobbies around the house, and group 3 the fewest of around-the-house activites (including TV watching). These differences tended to level off at age 25 when generally fewer hobbies and social activities were reported.

## 11. Delinquency

The relationship between LD, neurological impairment, and delinquency, as it appeared in the first Phase of the follow-up, has been described previously (Spreen 1981). Briefly, it was found that the presence of LD did not relate to an increased incidence of encounters with the police or to a greater number of offenses, although the LD group without neurological findings did receive a slightly higher number of somewhat more severe penalties than the neurologically impaired groups. The results of Phase I were clearly at variance with some prospective studies (Kirkegaard-Sorensen & Mednick 1977) and with retrospective studies which had described a close association between dropout rate and delinquency (Elliott 1984). Elliott did not find a relationship to social class, but did cite other contributing factors, such as experience with marriage and employment, and, for females, the home setting ('alienation') and social isolation. Other studies described a close association directly between LD and delinquency as well as between neurological dysfunction and delinquency (Berman 1978a, b; Berman & Siegal, 1976; Duling 1970; Pincus et al. 1979); Offord et al. (1978, 1983) viewed socio-familial variables and temperament as main factors, which he interpreted as etiologic for both LD and delinquency. The hypothesis that 'biological predisposition' towards criminality can be exacerbated by 'organic damage' (especially brain damage) or by 'cerebral birth trauma' has been presented by Christiansen (1977). In contrast, West and Farrington (1973), Mednick (1973) and Schulsinger (1976) reported that birth complications were not more frequently associated with delinquency. Herbst and Roesler (1986) reported higher delinquency rates for subjects who dropped out of school earlier or attended special school and who had unskilled jobs. They found no difference in IQ between delinquent and non-delinquent subjects, but the overall delinquency rate for subjects with perinatal damage was 21% compared to 4.2% for the same age range in East German statistics. The authors also computed a 'social risk index' correlation of .22 and a 'biological risk index' correlation of .36 with delinquency. Rutter and Giller (1983) expressed the view that brain damage has been shown to increase the risk of psychiatric disorder and educational retardation quite substantially and that, because of this link, it probably also increases the risk of delinquency (although

40

there is no direct association with delinquency). However, Vierkunen (Vierkunen & Nuutila 1976, Vierkunen et al. 1976) found some relationship between acquired brain damage and rate of delinquency.

The discrepancy between our results and other findings and interpretations is probably the result of the retrospective method of most studies (it is more likely that an association is found if a study starts with convicted offenders, but fails to follow peers with similar etiology who did not come to the attention of the police) as well as the interaction with socio-economic factors which were relatively homogeneous in our sample.

The age period covered in the Phase I interview coincides with the period of highest prevelance rates for convictions in general: The Cambridge Study of Delinquent Development (Farrington 1983) shows the highest rates between 13 and 17 years, a somewhat lower rate between 18 and 20, and a sharp drop after the age of 20. Similarly, Philips and Kelly (1979) and Elliott (1984) found that delinquency rates fall after school leaving. This has been interpreted as an association between delinquency and school failure which is no longer affecting the individual in the workplace after school.

The Phase I interview data were reanalyzed with the three LD groups matched for IQ. The reanalysis, however, basically confirmed our previous conclusions. The second follow-up covered additional encounters with the police, offenses and penalties received during the last 6 years. Phase I and Phase II data were then added for an analysis of the total record of each participant. It was noted earlier (Spreen 1981) that, in a comparison of parent and client interview, parents tended to report fewer incidents than clients. This was seen as an indication of the relative openness of our participants during the interview, suggesting that not many of them had actually misrepresented their delinquency record.

In both interviews, the 'opening question' was: 'Have you come to the attention of the police?'. Table 11-1 lists the percentage of yes responses to this question for Phase I and II. No significant difference between groups was found. There was also no significant sex difference, and no significant difference between groups for the age (median age 13) when the first encounter with the police occurred.

*Table 11-1: Percentage of Participants Coming to the Attention of the Police*

| Group | 1 | 2 | 3 | Control |
|---|---|---|---|---|
| Phase I (clients) | 53.8 | 52.2 | 58.8 | 57.7 |
| (parents) | 40.4 | 37.7 | 44.1 | 38.5 |
| Phase II (clients) | 38.5 | 40.5 | 42.6 | 48.6 |
| At both Phase I & II | | | | |
| Interviews | 31.3 | 31.5 | 28.6 | 45.1 |

41

The total number of offenses reported at Phase I and II are shown in Table 11-2. The difference between groups was not significant at both interviews, nor was the difference for the sum of offenses at both times significant.

*Table 11-2: Number of Offenses Reported at Phase I and II*

| Group | 1 | | 2 | | 3 | | Control | |
|---|---|---|---|---|---|---|---|---|
| Phase | I | II | I | II | I | II | I | II |
| no offense | 38.8 | 58.2 | 43.8 | 50.7 | 37.1 | 51.4 | 35.3 | 35.3 |
| 1 offense only | 37.3 | 17.9 | 26.0 | 13.7 | 34.3 | 17.1 | 31.4 | 35.3 |
| 2 offenses only | 7.5 | 6.0 | 15.1 | 6.8 | 8.6 | 11.4 | 15.7 | 7.8 |
| 3 offenses only | 6.0 | 4.5 | 5.5 | 8.2 | 8.6 | 8.6 | 11.8 | 11.8 |
| 4 or more offenses | 10.4 | 13.4 | 9.6 | 20.5 | 11.4 | 11.4 | 5.9 | 9.8 |

* The figures for Phase I differ slightly from those reported by Spreen (1981) because of changes in the population. In this table, both Phase I and Phase II figures are based on the same participants.

The types of offenses committed at both times are listed in Table 11-3. No significant overall differences were found at both times. However, one significant univariate difference was found for vehicle-moving offenses at the Phase I interview: the control subjects had more offenses of this type than the three LD groups ($p < .01$). This difference was probably due to the fact that more control group subjects started to drive at an earlier age. However, some of the difference was still present at the Phase II interview.

*Table 11-3: Percentage of Participants Reporting each*
*Type of Offense During Phase I and Phase II Interview*

| Group | 1 | | 2 | | 3 | | Control | |
|---|---|---|---|---|---|---|---|---|
| Phase | I | II | I | II | I | II | I | II |
| *Type of Offense* | | | | | | | | |
| Petty Crime | 17.5 | 7.5 | 11.0 | 1.4 | 2.9 | 2.9 | 13.7 | 3.9 |
| Property Violation | 22.4 | 9.0 | 11.0 | 4.1 | 14.3 | 2.9 | 5.9 | 4.9 |
| Person Violation | 3.0 | 1.5 | 1.4 | 0 | 5.7 | 5.7 | 0 | 2.0 |
| Drug Offenses | 11.9 | 7.5 | 8.2 | 0 | 14.3 | 0 | 2.0 | 0 |
| Vehicle Moving Offense | 16.4 | 28.4 | 19.2 | 41.1 | 28.4 | 31.4 | 49.0* | 48.2* |
| Routine Check, Looking Suspicious | 7.5 | 9.0 | 15.1 | 17.8 | 17.1 | 17.8 | 11.8 | 11.8 |
| Runaway, Truancy, Being Lost | 11.9 | 0 | 3.5 | 1.4 | 0 | 0 | 0 | 3.9 |
| Other | 6.0 | 0 | 1.4 | 0 | 2.9 | 0 | 5.9 | 0 |

* $p < .01$ at both interviews for vehicle-moving offenses (chi-square = 18.92 and 25.07).

42

Analyzing penalties reported during the Phase I interview, we found a significantly higher number of 'warnings' given to the subjects in groups 1 and 2. Deprivation of privileges was more often found in the control group, and licence suspensions occurred more often in Group 3 . The total number of minor penalties received during the second Phase of the follow-up did not differ significantly between groups. When penalties from both interviews were added, no significant group differences emerged for individual types of penalties (Table 11-4) nor for the total number of all penalties reported (Table 11-5).

*Table 11-4: Percentage of Participants Reporting Each Type of Penalty During Phase I and II Interviews*

| Group | 1 | | 2 | | 3 | | Control | |
|---|---|---|---|---|---|---|---|---|
| Phase | I | II | I | II | I | II | I | II |
| *Type of Penalty* | | | | | | | | |
| No Penalty or Charges, Acquittal | 26.9 | 16.4 | 27.4 | 11.0 | 31.4 | 2.9 | 27.5 | 3.9 |
| Warning, Talk to Parents | 20.9 | 22.4 | 12.3 | 38.4 | 2.9 | 25.7 | 11.8 | 54.9 |
| Deprivation of Privileges | 7.5 | 10.4 | 11.3 | 9.6 | 17.1 | 14.3 | 29.4 | 15.7 |
| Dollar Fine | 9.0 | 0 | 9.6 | 1.4 | 20.0 | 5.7 | 11.8 | 2.0 |
| Probation | 4.5 | 0 | 4.1 | 0 | 8.6 | 0 | 2.0 | 0 |
| Community Diversion, Community Work, Suspended Sentence | 1.5 | 4.5 | 4.1 | 2.7 | 5.7 | 11.4 | 0 | 2.0 |
| Prison | 3.0 | 3.0 | 2.7 | 6.8 | 8.6 | 17.1 | 0 | 4.9 |

chi-square $= 13.80, p < .31$

The offenses and penalties were broken down into minor and serious and reanalyzed. A significant difference between groups on serious offenses (property and person violations) was found more often in groups 1 and 3 (Table 11-6), although contrasting all three LD groups with controls did not produce a significant difference. The groups also differed on minor offenses (most frequent for the control group). There were no significant group differences for minor penalties received, but the difference for serious penalties for both interviews added together (Table 11-7) was significant. Groups 2 and 3 had 26 and 28 % of subjects who received such penalties, and the largest number of such penalties (long licence suspen-

Table 11-5: All Penalties Reported at Phase II Interview
by Group (in % of subjects in each group and % of the total
number of all penalties)

| Group | 1 | 2 | 3 | Control | Total |
|---|---|---|---|---|---|
| Zero | 29 | 25 | 9 | 18 | 81 |
| | 53.7 | 42.4 | 36.0 | 35.3 | |
| | 15.3 | 13.2 | 4.8 | 9.5 | |
| One | 13 | 10 | 6 | 20 | 49 |
| | 24.1 | 16.9 | 24.0 | 39.2 | |
| | 6.9 | 5.3 | 3.2 | 10.6 | |
| Two | 2 | 5 | 3 | 3 | 13 |
| | 3.7 | 8.5 | 12.0 | 5.9 | |
| | 1.1 | 2.6 | 1.6 | 1.6 | |
| Three | 4 | 6 | 3 | 5 | 18 |
| | 7.4 | 10.2 | 12.0 | 9.8 | |
| | 2.1 | 3.2 | 1.6 | 2.6 | |
| Four | 6 | 13 | 4 | 5 | 28 |
| | 11.1 | 22.0 | 16.0 | 9.8 | |
| | 3.2 | 6.9 | 2.1 | 2.6 | |
| | 54 | 59 | 25 | 51 | 189 |
| | 28.6 | 31.2 | 13.2 | 27.0 | 100.0 |

chi-square $= 13.80, p < .31$

sions, heavy fines, probation, community service, jail) were also found in groups 2 and 3, while only four subjects in the control group and one subject in group 1 received two of these penalties.

During the Phase II interview, sex offenses were specifically separated from other offenses. Only three subjects reported 1 sex offense, one reported 3, and one reported 4 such offenses. All five subjects were in the brain-damaged (Group 1) category. No conclusions regarding a relationship between sex offenses and LD can be drawn from this finding.

Intelligence level was not clearly related to delinquency. IQ scores were included in all analyses and checked for significance as covariates in an analysis of variance as well as for changes in the significance of contingency tables when these effects were controlled for. None of the covariance effects was significant; raw regression coefficients were in the order of .10 to .20. Partialling out the effect of VIQ, PIQ, and FSIQ changed the chi-square values only minimally. Observing (nonsignificant) trends, there was a tendency for subjects with lower IQs (70 to 88) to show a somewhat

Table 11-6: Frequency of Serious Offenses From Phase I and
Phase II Combined (Includes Property, Personal and Sexual Offenses)

| Group | 1 | 2 | 3 | Control | Total |
|-------|------|------|------|---------|-------|
| Zero | 32 | 50 | 18 | 46 | 146 |
| | 59.3 | 84.7 | 72.0 | 90.2 | |
| | 16.9 | 26.5 | 9.5 | 24.3 | |
| One | 14 | 6 | 1 | 3 | 24 |
| | 25.9 | 10.2 | 4.0 | 5.9 | |
| | 7.4 | 3.2 | 0.5 | 1.6 | |
| Two | 2 | 2 | 0 | 2 | 6 |
| | 3.7 | 3.4 | 0.0 | 3.9 | |
| | 1.1 | 1.1 | 0.0 | 1.1 | |
| Three | 4 | 0 | 4 | 0 | 8 |
| | 7.4 | 0.0 | 16.0 | 0.0 | |
| | 2.1 | 0.0 | 2.1 | 0.0 | |
| Four | 1 | 1 | 1 | 0 | 3 |
| | 1.9 | 1.7 | 4.0 | 0.0 | |
| | 0.5 | 0.5 | 0.5 | 0.0 | |
| Five | 1 | 0 | 1 | 0 | 2 |
| | 1.9 | 0.0 | 4.0 | 0.0 | |
| | 0.5 | 0.0 | 0.5 | 0.0 | |
| | 54 | 59 | 25 | 51 | 189 |
| | 28.6 | 31.2 | 13.2 | 27.0 | 100.0 |

chi-square $= 35.32, p < .002$

higher number of serious offenses, while, at the same time, subjects with higher IQs (110 and higher) tended to get slightly more serious penalties. However, the data do not allow more than speculation about such trends. Previous studies (Ensminger, Kellam, & Rubin 1983) showed significantly lower delinquency scores for subjects with low IQ while school readiness (Metropolitan Readiness score in grade 1) had only a moderate relation; however, the major relationship demonstrated in this project was between aggressiveness exhibited in grade 1 for both sexes, as well as high risk (change, single parent, nonintact) families at grade 1 (for boys only) and delinquency during the teenage years.

Sex differences indicated that males were more likely to report person violation and drug and alcohol offenses, and to receive jail sentences than females.

| Group | 1 | 2 | 3 | Control | Total |
|-------|------|------|------|---------|-------|
| Zero | 44 | 44 | 18 | 46 | 152 |
|      | 81.5 | 74.6 | 72.0 | 90.2 | |
| One | 6 | 6 | 1 | 4 | 17 |
|     | 11.1 | 10.2 | 4.0 | 7.8 | |
| Two | 1 | 4 | 0 | 1 | 6 |
|     | 1.9 | 6.8 | 0.0 | 2.0 | |
| Three | 1 | 3 | 1 | 0 | 5 |
|       | 1.9 | 5.1 | 4.0 | 0.0 | |
| Four | 1 | 2 | 1 | 0 | 4 |
|      | 1.9 | 3.4 | 4.0 | 0.0 | |
| Five | 1 | 0 | 3 | 0 | 4 |
|      | 1.9 | 0.0 | 12.0 | 0.0 | |
| Six | 0 | 0 | 1 | 0 | 1 |
|     | 0.0 | 0.0 | 4.0 | 0.0 | |
|     | 54 | 59 | 25 | 51 | 189 |
|     | 28.6 | 31.2 | 13.2 | 27.0 | 100.0 |

chi-square $= 31.35, p < .026$

One other relationship, namely between hyperactivity between the ages of 4 and 12 years (interpreted by the authors as evidence of minimal brain damage) and later delinquency and drug abuse, has been reported by Loney, Whaley-Klahn, Kosier and Conboy (1983). This topic will be explored in Section 22.

In *summary*, the results of Phase II of the follow-up bear out the contention that a history of LD as such does not increase the incidence of offenses of any particular type to a significant degree, although some of our subgroups of LD reported more serious offenses, while the control group committed more minor offenses. As found in our earlier analysis, subjects in the LD group without identifiable brain dysfunction and with suspected brain dysfunction received more and more serious penalties, although this difference - compared to the control group - was not significant when all three LD groups were pooled and the comparison repeated.

## 12. Assistance Sought and Received

Information about specialists and other helping professionals consulted or employed ranged from tutoring and special education teachers to specialists in audiology and psychiatry.

During the first interview, a significant difference between groups was found for the question whether the participants had seen a physician for any type of problem (100, 95.1, 80.0, 89.1% for groups 1 to 4 respectively; chi-square $= 13.25, p < .004$). No significant group differences were found when asked whether other physicians or specialists were consulted, and whether they saw speech and hearing specialists. The LD groups were more often seen by a psychiatrist or psychologist (51.6, 44.3, 44.1 vs. 9.8%; chi-square $= 23.74, p < .001$), by an educational or vocational counsellor (29.5, 13.9, 36.4 vs. 2.0%; chi-square $= 21.78, p < .0011$), and by additional professionals for advice on his/her problem (37.3, 11.7, 22.2 vs. 6.4%; chi-square $= 19.37, p < .0002$).

An analysis of Phase II follow-up questions indicates that groups 1 and 2 consulted more specialists, and that a single specialist (Table 12-1) was most frequently consulted by our control group. However, this difference appears to be due to a few subjects who contacted a larger variety of specialists. The analysis of types of specialists by group provided no significant group differences except for psychological and psychiatric consultation. A repeat analysis with IQ-matched groups came to almost identical results.

Table 12-1: Percent of Participants Consulting Specialists
at Phase II Interview (Includes Ophthalmology, ENT, Optometry,
Audiology, Speech Pathology)

|  | Group 1 | Group 2 | Group 3 | Control |
|---|---|---|---|---|
| none | 52 | 53 | 68 | 29 |
| one specialist | 42 | 38 | 29 | 66 |
| two | 6 | 7 | 3 | 4 |
| three | 0 | 1 | 0 | 0 |
|  | chi-square $= 18.43, p < .030$ | | | |

A separate set of questions addressed the consultation of psychology or psychiatry specialists. However, for the Phase II period neither the total number of consultations nor the total for either profession was significantly different between groups. There was a trend, however, for LD participants to consult psychiatrists more often (16.7% of group 1, 18.5% of group 2, 12.5% of group 3, and 7.4% of group 4). The results remained unchanged when the analysis was repeated with IQ-matched groups.

Table 12-2 shows the consultation of educational or vocational counsellors mentioned in the Phase II interview. The difference between groups relies mainly on the younger participants who had not had vocational or educational counselling prior to the Phase I interview.

Table 12-2: Consultation with Educational or
Vocational Counsellors (in %)

|  | Group 1 | Group 2 | Group 3 | Control |
|---|---|---|---|---|
| no consultation | 55 | 66 | 84 | 86 |
| voluntary | 31 | 29 | 4 | 14 |
| mandatory | 14 | 5 | 12 | 0 |

chi-square $= 22.06, p < .001$

None of the analyses of assistance sought and received showed a significant difference between male and female participants.

The high variability of treatment variables is, of course, due to the fact that our participants came from many different schools and school districts with differing resources, and the additional help parents may or may not find from private sources such as summer school, tutoring, private schools, and tutoring services, as well as in counselling.

Section 26 will explore the various intervention and treatment variables by first forming factors of treatment, and then relating these to the major factors of outcome. ·

In *summary*, the LD groups were more often seen by psychiatrists or psychologists, or by vocational or educational counsellors. Other intervention and treatment variables will be discussed in section 26.

# b. Repeat Examination and Questions of Long-term Stability

### 13. Neurological Examination

The neurological examination included findings on 26 separate examinations or test observations made by the neurologist. These range from checks of eye movement and muscle tone to reflexes and observations of physical asymmetries. Because of their diversity, a meaningful grouping of neurological signs may be expected to yield better results than a mere summary score. In addition, the degree of impairment on each check was described as normal, slightly impaired and marked (see Appendix 5).

Neurological soft signs have been considered by some as age-related or 'maturational', unreliable, or of no importance in the neurological evaluation of the child (Adams et al. 1974; Greenberg & McMahon 1977; Schmitt 1975). Poor cognitive abilities, inattention, and poor motivation have also been suggested as possible 'causes'. Other authors, however, (Ackerman et al. 1977a; Hertzig et al. 1968 & 1969) view soft signs as indicators of a compromised nervous system of uncertain etiology which may persist past middle childhood. Few studies have addressed the issue of the persistence of soft signs directly, and those that have (Peters et al. 1975; Hertzig et al. 1968 & 1969) report mixed results. A study by Menkes, Rowe, and Menkes (1967), though based on only 14 subjects with LD and hyperactivity, reported more subjects with neurological dysfunction at follow-up than at intake, and suggested a 'trend towards worsening or at least crystallization of neurological symptoms, rather than resolution' (Helper 1980) of the neurological status. Herbst and Roesler (1986) found 14.6% of their subjects with perinatal and congenital impairment to have abnormal neurological findings; 55.3% had abnormal EEGs, and 42.5% abnormal x-ray findings. On repeat examination in adulthood there was no change in neurological status (although the correlation was only .41), but abnormal EEGs were present only in 30.7%.

The current study addressed the issue of persistence of both hard and soft signs, both as a direct matter of study as well as a major variable related to long-term outcome, the main purpose of the project. A neurological reexamination was conducted with all participants including control subjects during the Phase II evaluation.. While the neurological examination at the time of first referral was conducted for almost all LD participants by two neurologists, the Phase II examination was conducted by the project neurologist who was 'blind' to group classification and previous neurological findings, and who did not take a history of the participants but who had seen a substantial number of the clients at referral age. The average time elapsed between first and second neurological assessment was 13.9 years (Hern & Spreen 1984).

*Table 13-1: Percentage of Subjects in Each Group Showing*
*Hard and Soft Signs at Referral Age (Time 1)*
*and Phase II (Time 2)*

|  | Hard Signs | | Soft Signs | |
|---|---|---|---|---|
|  | Time 1 | Time 2 | Time 1 | Time 2 |
| Group 1 | 100% | 54.8% | 100% | 93.5% |
| Group 2 | 0% | 23.9% | 100% | 84.8% |
| Group 3 | 0% | 11.8% | 0% | 72.5% |

The percentages of subjects in the three LD groups with hard and soft signs at referral age and Phase II (Table 13-1) suggest that there is little improvement in the neurological status of LD subjects over this period. Soft signs show some improvement in the original neurologically impaired groups, but strikingly, group 3, which had no neurological findings at referral age, now shows a large number of such signs. There is a significant increase also in hard signs. The breakdown into three IQ levels shown in Figure 13-1 and 13-2 indicates that there is little change in hard signs for the low IQ group, and some improvement in the highest IQ group. A regression analysis indicates a significant relationship between intake and Phase II neurological examination summed scores ($F[1,121] = 134.48; p < .001$, corresponding to a correlation coefficient of .73). The greatest increase is seen in the middle IQ groups (IQ level effect $F(2, 107) = 1.29; p < .28$; Time effect $F = 5.35; p < .02$; Time x IQ $F = 0.46; p < .63$). However, there was an IQ effect for soft signs, related to the overall increase in soft signs (IQ effect $F(3, 116) = 5.73$; p < .001; Time effect $F = 70.70; p < .001$; Time x IQ $F = 2.38; p < .07$) (Hern 1984).

The control group had no hard signs. The IQ variable for this group does not extend into the lower end and hence cannot be compared with the three LD groups. However, if IQ levels 3 (91-105) and 4 (106-120) are analyzed separately, a significant group effect and no IQ effect can be found.

Each of the neurological functions was analyzed separately: 9 out of 26 showed significant deterioration, 11 showed no change, and only 2 (choreiform/athetoid movement, incoordination) showed improvement (Table 13-2).

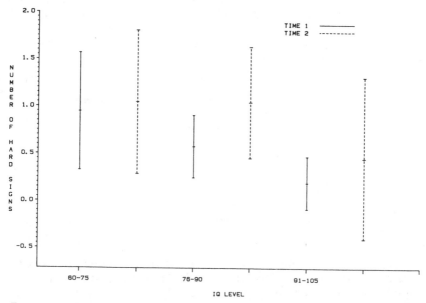

*Figure 13-1: Number of Hard Neurological Signs at Time 1 and 2 by IQ level*

50

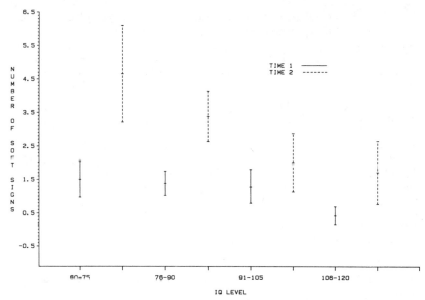

*Figure 13-2: Number of Soft Neurological Signs at Time 1 and 2 by IQ level*

Only four of the soft signs were found in more than two members of the control group. When these four signs were analyzed with respect to differences between LD and control groups, significant differences remained for all but one sign.

The findings contradict the notion that soft signs are maturational and disappear as the person grows up. Correlations between time 1 and time 2 are of moderate size, suggesting persistence over the follow-up period, and thus lend support to the earlier findings by Menkes, Rowe, and Menkes (1967) and Herbst and Roesler (1986). The significance of such signs as well as that of hard signs is, of course, explored in the main body of this report.

A review of the neurological examination was undertaken to check how many of our participants had lateralized signs at the Phase II examination. While 56 of the subjects had no lateralization, 21 were found to have findings pointing towards right-hemisphere localization, and 56 left-hemisphere localization. In a comparison of achievement test data (WRAT, PIAT, WAIS-Arith) at Phase II between right- and left-hemisphere groups, no significant multivariate or univariate differences were found.

Right- and left-hemisphere groups also did not differ when a comparison of the frequency of occurrence of each of nine LD clusters (see Section 21) was attempted, nor did they differ between the four categories used throughout this monograph. It would seem that for the variables analyzed so far, and for the relatively small number of participants for whom

51

Table 13-2: Percent Change in Neurological Signs in Three LD
Groups from Referral Age to Age 25 (Phase II)

| Neurological Sign | Group 1 | | | Group 2 | | | Group 3 | | |
|---|---|---|---|---|---|---|---|---|---|
| | Ties* | Better | Worse | Ties | Better | Worse | Ties | Better | Worse |
| Ataxia | 52% | 10% | 39%& | 77% | 7% | 16% | 87% | - | 13%* |
| Asymmetry of skull or limbs | 61 | 6 | 32 * | 61 | 2 | 36 & | 90 | - | 10 * |
| Visual field defect | 90 | 3 | 6 | 100 | - | - | 100 | - | - |
| Diplopia | 94 | 3 | 3 | 100 | - | - | 98 | - | 2 |
| Strabismus | 77 | 3 | 19 | 95 | 2 | 2 | 100 | - | - |
| Nystagmus | 90 | 3 | 6 | 100 | - | - | 100 | - | - |
| Dysarthria | 58 | 6 | 36 & | 73 | 2 | 25 & | 100 | - | - |
| Dyspraxia of tongue movement | 77 | 6 | 16 | 95 | 2 | 2 | 100 | - | - |
| Choreiform, athetoid movements | 52 | 23 | 26 | 70 | 30 | - & | 98 | - | 2 |
| Resting muscle tone | 58 | 19 | 23 | 73 | 2 | 25 . & | 92 | - | 8 |
| Paresis | 58 | . 13 | 29 | 91 | - | 9 | 98 | - | 2 |
| Diminished/hyper-active tendon reflexes | 45 | 13 | 42 | 59 | 7 | 34 & | 75 | - | 25 & |
| Babinski sign | 77 | 8 | 13 | 84 | - | 16 & | 94 | - | 6 |
| Incoordination | 45 | 39 | 16 | 55 | 36 | 9 & | 85 | - | 15 & |
| Heel/knee test | 48 | 19 | 32 | 84 | - | 16 & | 92 | - | 8 |
| Disdiadochokinesia | 45 | 3 | 52 & | 75 | 7 | 18 | 98 | - | 2 |
| Anaesthesia | 84 | 6 | 10 | 95 | 5 | - | 100 | - | - |
| Simultagnosia | 84 | 13 | 3 | 100 | - | - | 98 | - | 2 |
| Graphaesthesia | 55 | 13 | 32 | 68 | 18 | 14 | 85 | - | 15 & |

* Ties = No change
* $p < .05$ (2-tailed test)
& $p < .01$ (2-tailed test)

lateralization data were available, no meaningful difference between right and left cortical localization in terms of functions is indicated. It should be noted that the literature dealing with lateralization of function is almost entirely based on acquired and severe cortical damage. Lateralization of mild degree or minimal neurological signs of early perinatal origin are not necessarily expected to replicate these findings.

In order to reanalyze some of our findings with a more meaningful subscore of the neurological examination, four signs were disregarded because of their extremely low frequency of occurrence, and the remaining 22 subjected to a principal component factor analysis. The results (Table 13-3) suggested the following groupings of neurological signs which have been labelled for ease of description according to the main neurological system or systems involved:

factor 1: motor: ataxia, resting tremor, muscle tone, paresis, incoordination, heel-knee test, disdiadochokinesis, intention tremor.

factor 2: sensory: graphesthesia, anesthesia, position sense, simultagnosia.

factor 3: motor/speech: dysarthria, dyspraxia of tongue, choreoform movements.

factor 4: visual: nystagmus, strabismus.

factor 5: motor/peripheral/asymmetry: asymmetry of skull and limb, tendon reflexes, clonus, Babinski sign.

The grouping into these factors was also accepted on the basis of an inspection of the intercorrelation matrix and because they form clinically meaningful groups of symptoms.

Using the rating of 1 (abnormal), 2 (slight abnormality) and 3 (normal), these factors can now be used in the form of (a) sums for each factor, or (b) weighted factor scores, in further analyses.

Using sum scores for each factor, we investigated the stability of neuro-

Table 13-3: Rotated Factors of 22 Neurological Signs

| Sign | Factor | | | | |
|---|---|---|---|---|---|
| | 1 | 2 | 3 | 4 | 5 |
| ataxia | 55 | 35 | 37 | 31 | 20 |
| asymmetry | 00 | 64 | 16 | 04 | -07 |
| strabismus | 13 | 29 | 07 | 76 | 00 |
| nystagmus | 12 | 15 | 00 | 66 | 00 |
| dysarthria | 20 | 26 | 75 | 02 | 17 |
| dyspraxia | 17 | 03 | 81 | 06 | -12 |
| choreoform movements | 57 | 00 | 63 | 03 | 10 |
| resting tremor | 69 | 24 | -12 | -18 | -11 |
| muscle tone | 50 | 61 | 21 | 33 | 09 |
| paresis | 57 | 50 | 12 | 34 | 12 |
| tendon reflexes | 44 | 59 | 20 | 23 | 13 |
| ancle clonus | 47 | 64 | 00 | 13 | 13 |
| Babinski | 30 | 57 | 00 | 34 | 01 |
| synkinesis | 08 | 38 | 40 | -03 | 14 |
| incoordination | 75 | 17 | 28 | 33 | 16 |
| heel-knee test | 75 | 24 | 26 | 36 | 15 |
| intention tremor | 67 | 07 | 25 | 00 | -04 |
| disdiadochokinesis | 70 | 19 | 39 | 23 | 16 |
| anaesthesia | 07 | 19 | 08 | 12 | 74 |
| simultagnosia | 00 | -25 | -04 | 04 | 75 |
| position sense | 37 | 32 | 00 | -38 | 49 |
| graphaesthesia | 03 | 19 | 00 | -38 | 49 |

logical signs in more detail. Table 13-4 shows the sum scores for each factor at the first and second neurological examination as well as the results of a repeated-measures MANOVA analysis. The analyses allow a more detailed look at the stability of neurological signs: while the overall stability is highly significant (canonical correlation = .540), only the signs summed under factors 1, 4, and 5 show a significant change, while the signs summed under factor 2 (sensory) do not change significantly and the signs under factor 3 (speech) only marginally.

*Table 13-4: Sums of Neurological Sign Groups at First and Second Examination*

|  | Neurological Examination | |
| --- | --- | --- |
| *Factor* | First | Second |
| 1 Motor | 22.9 | 21.6 |
| 2 Sensory | 11.7 | 11.7 |
| 3 Motor/Speech | 8.7 | 8.5 |
| 4 Visual | 5.9 | 5.8 |
| 5 Motor/Peripheral/Asymmetry | 11.6 | 10.6 |

Repeated measure manova: $F = 10.21, p < .001$
univariate $F$s  Factor 1   $= 26.96, p < .001$
           Factor 2   $= 1.02, p < .314$
           Factor 3   $= 3.19, p < .076$
           Factor 4   $= 5.33, p < .023$
           Factor 5   $= 48.17, p < .001$

Other analyses using the grouping of neurological signs were conducted using factor-weighted scores rather than sum scores for each factor. These analyses are reported in the sections on achievement tests (14) and subtypes of LD (21).

In *summary*, our LD population was divided into groups with hard neurological signs, soft signs, and no neurological findings, based on the referral-age examination. Neurological reexamination at age 25 indicated little improvement in neurological status in groups 1 and 2, but group 3 also showed now a large number of soft signs and a moderate number of hard signs. Correlation between the two neurological examinations overall was .73. Increased neurological signs were found for the subjects in the middle range of IQ, not for the high- and low-IQ participants. Only choreoform/athetoid movement and incoordination were found less frequently at adult age. Lateralization of signs indicating right or left hemisphere dysfunction was not related to achievement test results or subtype of LD. The neurological signs were factor-analyzed to form 5 factors useful for further analysis of meaningful groups of signs in later sections. Significant changes from the first to the second neurological examination were noted only for signs grouped as factor 1 (motor), factor 4 (visual), and factor 5 (motor/peripheral/asymmetry).

## 14. Achievement Tests

By definition, our LD subjects were poor in at least one area of school achievement at the time of the original referral. Subtracting the grade level expected on the basis of age at the time of testing from the actual class grade at that time, group 1 subjects were an average of 1.57 years behind expectation, group 2 subjects an average of 1.5, and group 3 subjects an average of 1.17. Their reading level (WRAT) at that time was an average of 1.53, .80, and .86 years below the level expected on the basis of age alone. In spelling (WRAT), they were 1.83, 1.42, and 1.22 grades behind, in arithmetic (WRAT) 2.09, 1.68, and 1.20 grades behind. The difference between LD groups was statistically significant. By definition, our control group performed at grade level or better. Experience with this particular test (WRAT, 1978 version) in the Western British Columbia suggests that this lag is an under-estimate, since during the early elementary grades test scores in this area tend to be almost a full year higher than the expected grade level (McAllister & Spreen 1981).

The difference between the three LD groups after matching for IQ (see Section 24) was not significant for the achievement test results nor for achievement corrected for grade level, although the direction of differences was still present (WRAT Reading 1.42, 0.92, and 0.38).

It is of special interest how academic achievement proceeded from that level during the course of the school career of our LD participants. The following analyses were conducted to investigate whether these children fell further behind or whether they were able to catch up during their school years or during their early adult life.

Participants in group 1 completed an average of 10.09 grades (see section 7). The number of grades completed for group 2 was 10.53, for group 3 10.42, and for the control group 11.96 ($F$ [3, 185]; $p < .001$).

The Phase II tests included the WRAT and the Peabody Individual Achievement Test (PIAT) (Reading Comprehension) as measures of current abilities in reading, spelling, and arithmetic. In addition, the WAIS-R arithmetic subtest provides an estimate of our participants' ability to handle verbally encoded arithmetic problems. A striking difference in all achievement areas between the three LD groups and our control group was noted. Table 14-1 shows that our control group was able to read (word recognition) at a level equivalent to grade 10 while all three LD groups were at the grade 7 level. Within the three LD groups, a linear trend was noted with the poorest reading in group 1 and the best reading in group 3, although the differences were small. A similar difference between LD and control subjects and, in this case more pronounced, between LD groups was found for PIAT reading comprehension scores (also in school grade level equivalents). The test has a ceiling of grade 12.9, so that it can be inferred that many control group subjects performed at or near ceiling level for this test.

*Table 14-1: Mean WRAT Reading and PIAT Reading Comprehension Grade Scores (n in brackets)*

| Group | 1 | 2 | 3 | Control |
|---|---|---|---|---|
| WRAT Reading | 7.32 | 7.42 | 7.78 | 10.29 |
| | ( 53) | ( 59) | ( 26) | ( 49) |
| PIAT Reading Comp. | 7.95 | 9.18 | 9.90 | 12.32 |
| | ( 51) | ( 59) | ( 26) | ( 51) |

| | |
|---|---|
| WRAT Reading | $F(3) = 26.19, p < .001$ |
| PIAT Reading Comprehension | $F(3) = 18.79, p < .001$ |

The difference between the three LD groups is, however, highly dependent on IQ. A reanalysis of both the PIAT and the WRAT reading scores at the Phase II testing produced no significant differences between these three groups matched for IQ on a multiple range test (PIAT: grade 9.22, 9.47, and 10.41; WRAT Reading: grade 7.35, 7.43, and 8.01). These figures also suggest that in former LD subjects reading comprehension is better than the reading of individual new words ('word attack') as measured by the WRAT. Differences in the standardization samples of the two tests may be in part responsible for the difference, but cannot explain the full difference of almost two grades.

Spelling (WRAT) showed a similar significant group difference. The control group was about three full grade levels higher than the LD groups (Table 14-2). The three LD groups were not significantly different when matched for IQ (WRAT Spelling: Grade 6.81, 6.08, and 6.58).

*Table 14-2: Mean WRAT Spelling and Arithmetic Grade Levels (n in brackets)*

| Group | 1 | 2 | 3 | Control |
|---|---|---|---|---|
| WRAT Spelling | 6.06 | 5.86 | 6.29 | 9.90 |
| | ( 54) | ( 59) | ( 26) | ( 49) |
| WRAT Arithmetic | 5.07 | 5.22 | 5.25 | 8.43 |
| | ( 54) | ( 59) | ( 26) | ( 48) |
| WAIS Arithmetic | 7.64 | 7.40 | 7.56 | 11.44 |
| | ( 54) | ( 59) | ( 26) | ( 48) |

| | |
|---|---|
| WRAT Spelling | $F(3) = 35.10, p < .001$ |
| WRAT Arithmetic | $F(3) = 39.32, p < .001$ |
| WAIS Arithmetic | $F(3) = 38.52, p < .001$ |

Arithmetic (WRAT) also showed the three LD groups approximately three grade levels behind the control group (Table 14-2). After matching for IQ, the three LD groups were not significantly different, although the trend in the results remained (grade level 5.97, 5.34, and 5.34 respectively). The WAIS-R arithmetic scores are not in grade level terms, but in standard scores with a mean of 10. Our control group performed these verbally encoded arithmetic tasks at a high average and the three LD groups at a significantly below average level. The comparison of the three IQ-matched LD groups did not show significant differences (scaled scores: 9.09, 7.78, 7.54 respectively).

None of the results on achievement tests had significant differences between male and female participants.

A multivariate analysis included the test results during the Phase II examination, at the time of the original referral as well as the number of school grades completed, and the class grade at the time of referral. Because of the varying age at the time of the original referral, achievement test scores at that time were corrected according to the 'expected grade', i.e., these scores reflect the difference between expected grade and grade level obtained during testing.

Table 14-3: Factor Analysis of Achievement Tests and School
Grades Completed at Initial Referral and at Phase II Testing

|  | Factor 1 | Factor 2 | Factor 3 | Factor 4 |
|---|---|---|---|---|
| *Referral Age Tests* | | | | |
| WISC - Arithmetic | .10222 | .22329 | .31327 | .81876 |
| WRAT - Reading | .69573 | .33116 | .50511 | .03405 |
| WRAT - Spelling | .70224 | .27191 | .58280 | .02530 |
| WRAT - Arithmetic | .15372 | .37089 | .79574 | .24985 |
| Class Grade | .19077 | .23250 | .86909 | .01623 |
| *Phase II Tests* | | | | |
| Grades Completed | -.01983 | .62950 | .09449 | .02937 |
| WRAT - Reading | .55352 | .76666 | .13354 | .07757 |
| WRAT - Spelling | .60023 | .71431 | .13303 | .08440 |
| WRAT - Arithmetic | .06026 | .74356 | .35759 | .37818 |
| WAIS - Arithmetic | .09195 | .72309 | .36805 | .28570 |
| PIAT - Reading Compre. | .36946 | .63972 | .22753 | .12552 |
| *Referral Age Tests* | | | | |
| *Corrected for Age* | | | | |
| WISC - Arithmetic | .22383 | .12527 | -.09299 | .94890 |
| WRAT - Reading | .93332 | .13760 | .02378 | .15968 |
| WRAT - Spelling | .94975 | .06193 | .06767 | .17213 |
| WRAT - Arithmetic | .53099 | .16006 | .10254 | .55106 |
| Class Grade | .67852 | .11329 | .26281 | .26054 |

Table 14-3 presents a factor analysis of these results. Factor 1 clearly reflects a reading factor including all types of reading achievement at both times. Factor 2 seems to reflect mainly the scores obtained during Phase II testing, and factor 3 the results of initial referral tests. Factor 4 is a residual factor with loadings representing mainly the arithmetic tasks. It is of interest to note that the two types of academic skills show relative independence in factor analysis.

A canonical correlation attempted to investigate the relationship between achievement test results in young adulthood and neurological signs grouped as factors as described in section 13. This analysis should indicate which, if any, of the neurological findings have the greatest bearing on achievement test outcome. In contrast to the factor analysis reported above, the achievement test factors in this canonical analysis only used the Phase II measures and did not include the referral-age results. Only one significant canonical correlation was found ($r = .377, p < .0051$) between the first neurological examination factor described above ('motor') and the first achievement test factor (a general achievement factor with loadings on all tests). The standardized canonical coefficients indicated that this factor relied mainly on the reading rather than the arithmetic measures.

While the relationship found in this analysis is relatively weak, albeit significant, it indicates that all measures of reading are positively related to motor integrity, even at the adult age.

In *summary*, our LD subjects were on average between 1 and 2 years behind the school achievement level expected on the basis of age. At age 25, control subjects performed at a grade 10 level or better on tests of reading, spelling, and arithmetic, while the LD groups scored approximately 2 1/2 grades or more below them. Reading comprehension was generally better than reading of individual words ('word attack'). IQ accounted for part of the slow academic development, but even after IQ-matching the LD groups lagged considerably behind. Class grade and achievement test scores were factor analyzed and formed 3 meaningful factors, a reading factor, a factor representing referral age measures, and a factor representing adult re-test results. Relating achievement test results with groupings of neurological findings was achieved only for the 'motor' factor which was significantly related to a general achievement (reading) factor ($r = .377$).

### 15. Intelligence Tests

Few studies have repeated intelligence tests after a long time period. For a population of 27 subjects similar to ours, Herbst and Roesler (1986) found a striking consistency of IQ-test results over a 10-year period. Mean IQs were 96.26 at first testing and 95.82 10 years later, VIQs were 94.39 and

92.68, and PIQs were 96.58 and 98.65 respectively, using a German version of the Wechsler Intelligence Test ($r = .78$). The authors stressed that these results were strongly related to SES and other environmental variables.

The WISC-R was administered at referral age and the WAIS-R at the Phase II examination. Each individual subtest as well as the IQ-scores were analyzed for group and sex differences. At time 1, only the WISC Similarities subtest (Group means 9.2, 10.8, and 11.6 respectively), the Vocabulary subtest (means 9.3, 10.6, and 11.9), Picture Completion (means 10.0, 11.1, 12.0), Picture Arrangement (means 7.8, 9.8, and 11.1), Object Assembly (8.7, 10.1, 10.8) and Coding (6.7, 8.3, and 9.9) showed significant differences between the three LD groups. The VIQ difference between groups at Time 1 was significant at the .02 level (means 90.6, 95.8, 99.4), while the PIQ difference was highly significant (.001) (means 89.6, 97.9, 104.9). No significant sex differences or sex by group interactions were found.

At Phase II, significant group differences were found for the following subtests: Information (7.1, 7.6, 7.9 and 10.4), Digit Span (6.8, 7.6, 7.6, and 10.75), Vocabulary (7.3, 7.8, 8.2, and 11.3), Arithmetic (see Section 14), Comprehension (7.9, 8.8, 9.15, and 12.2), Similarities (7.2, 8.1, 8.6, and 11.6), Picture Completion (8.1, 9.7, 10.7, and 11.5), Picture Arrangement (8.2, 9.9, 9.8, and 11.8), Block Design (8.0, 9.0, 9.5, and 11.9), Object Assembly (7.1, 8.7, 9.1, and 10.4), and Digit Symbol (6.3, 7.3, 7.6, and 11.5). None of the sex differences were significant, although for WAIS Picture Arrangement a sex-by-group interaction was found. It can be seen that the group differences are significant mainly because of the good test results of the control group, but that in general a trend towards poorest results for group 1 and towards better results in group 3 persists in the second testing, suggesting a persisting effect of brain damage on skill development in these areas. All group differences on subtests remained significant after matching of groups for IQ.

The overall IQ scores differ appropriately: The WAIS-R VIQ was significantly different between groups (84.9, 87.6, 89.0, and 108.8), as was the PIQ (84.1, 91.8, 94.6, 109.7) and the Full-Scale IQ (83.1, 88.3, 90.5, and 110.3). After matching the LD groups for IQ the difference between LD groups and controls remained significant (89.65, 90.08, 91.79, and 110.27 respectively). No significant sex differences were found.

Considerations about the lateralization of lesions in at least a portion of LD children has led to speculations that either the verbal or the visuo-spatial abilities should be relatively more impaired. Hence a VIQ - PIQ discrepancy on the WISC or WAIS has been postulated by some authors (Black 1974; Klonoff & Low 1974), usually favoring VIQ, although several other authors failed to find such a difference (see discussion by Filskov and Leli 1981). Recently, Page and Steffi (1984) reported an average VIQ-PIQ difference of +5.40 with schizophrenic, neurotic, and personality-disorder patients on the WAIS. VIQ was higher for males, although the difference score was not significantly affected by sex or diagnosis. The authors pointed out that this finding contradicts the left-hemisphere-deficit hypothesis for schizophrenia (Flor-Henry 1976; Tucker 1981) which would lead to the expectation of a lower VIQ. For nonpsychotic children with emotional and behaviour difficulties, the authors found a mean difference score of -4.60 on the WISC-R.

An attempt was made to analyze the differences between VIQ and PIQ at both referral age and at Phase II follow-up. This analysis showed only one significant contrast between Groups 1, 2, and 3 for the difference score at Phase II retest, suggesting a somewhat higher VIQ in the brain-damaged group compared to other LD adults. No significant differences were found for the absolute difference scores at both times and for the actual difference at referral age (Table 15-1). The analyses remained nonsignificant with IQ-matched groups. It should be noted that even the largest absolute mean difference (13.3 points) is still within the range shown by 84.5% of the Wechsler normative sample (Matarazzo & Herman 1984). Where major differences do appear, the largest difference occurs in group 3 (LD without neurological findings). Such a finding is contrary to expectations, i.e., that the brain-damaged group would show the largest discrepancy between the two IQ scores. The heterogeneity of the sample in terms of VIQ-PIQ differences is expressed in the high standard deviations. However, using absolute difference scores does not bring out a more significant finding.

A final analysis of the VIQ-PIQ difference was made with the assumption that, although the actual mean score was not significantly different between groups both at referral and adult age, the brain-damaged groups have an exceptionally large number of individuals with large VIQ-PIQ differences. To test this, the VIQ-PIQ difference scores were broken down into high negative, medium (within + or − 10) and high positive range scores according to suitable breakpoints along the total score distribution. A chi-square analysis between the four groups and the three score-distribution levels was not significant at referral age, but reached significance ($p < .04$) at adult age. Group 1 contained more middle-range and high positive scorers, and group 4 (controls) had more extreme scorers at both ends of the distribution, while groups 2 and 3 had more subjects in the middle and high negative score range. The finding is not consistent with expectations, and should, in the absence of other positive findings, not be used for speculation without replication.

In *summary*, the three LD groups differed in IQ scores as well as in scores on several subtests both at the time of referral and at age 25. After matching for FSIQ, the subtest differences between groups remained significant. We found little support for an expected VIQ-PIQ discrepancy in LD children in either direction or in absolute values, except for the contrast of group 1 with groups 2 and 3. Searching for individuals with

a) *Referral Age (WISC-R)*

| Group | 1 | 2 | 3 | $p<$ |
|---|---|---|---|---|
| *n* | 58 | 69 | 31 | |
| $\overline{V}$IQ | 90.1 | 95.8 | 100.0 | |
| *SD* | 16.1 | 13.4 | 15.5 | |
| PIQ | 89.8 | 98.5 | 105.5 | |
| *SD* | 16.1 | 14.2 | 14.7 | |
| VIQ-PIQ | 0.35 | -2.65 | -5.42 | .2 |
| *SD* | 14.5 | 12.7 | 15.0 | |
| male | 0.98 | -3.96 | -3.90 | |
| female | -1.64 | 1.06 | -8.18 | |
| overall male-female | -2.19 vs. | -2.06 | n.s | |
| VIQ-PIQ(abs.)* | 11.9 | 10.2 | 13.2 | .22 |
| *SD* | 8.1 | 7.9 | 8.7 | |

b) *Phase II (WAIS-R)*

| Group | 1 | 2 | 3 | 4 | $p<$ |
|---|---|---|---|---|---|
| *n* | 54 | 59 | 26 | 51 | |
| VIQ | 84.9 | 87.6 | 89.0 | 108.8 | |
| *SD* | 14.3 | 11.3 | 13.3 | 11.9 | |
| PIQ | 84.1 | 91.8 | 94.6 | 109.7 | |
| *SD* | 15.1 | 12.9 | 12.0 | 10.1 | |
| VIQ-PIQ | .78 | -4.2 | -5.6 | -.88 | .03 |
| *SD* | 11.3 | 9.2 | 11.6 | 11.9 | |
| male | 1.02 | -2.8 | -6.0 | .2 | |
| female | -0.0 | -8.6 | -4.8 | -2.6 | n.s. |
| overall male-female: -1.8 vs. -4.6 | | | | | n.s. |
| VIQ-PIQ(abs.)* | 8.1 | 7.9 | 10.0 | 9.8 | .36 |
| *SD* | 7.8 | 6.2 | 7.9 | 6.6 | |

* abs. = absolute values

high discrepancy scores, group 1 showed more subjects with high VIQ, and group 2 and 3 more subjects with high and middle range PIQ.

## 16. Lateral Dominance over Time

The pattern of handedness in LD children has been the subject of much debate, speculation, and investigation with contradictory results. Usually, LD children in clinic-referred samples are more likely to show higher than average rates of nondextrality while poor learners in school samples often do not confirm these findings. Different measures of lateralization also do not necessarily form a unitary dimension (Eling 1983). Reports also indicate that in populations with neuropathology, such as epileptics and retardates, the incidence of left-handedness is at least twice as high as in the normal population. This excess of left-handedness is considered an indicator of pathology; neuropathology is assumed to have led to a switch in natural (genetic) handedness. Higher rates in clinic-referred samples may suggest higher incidence of neuropathology. In our population, an increase in nondextrality was expected to occur as a function of degree of neurological impairment.

At the time of referral, our subjects were given a questionnaire concerning their manual preference for each of seven tasks. If any doubt about the validity of a child's response existed, the child was asked to demonstrate the activity in question. Subjects were also given a test of grip strength (Dynamometer) and asked to write their name with each hand to allow an evaluation of the relative performance advantage. The same tests were administered at adult follow-up. Because of inconsistencies in test selection and subject attrition, 102 subjects received all three tests at time of referral, 124 at adult testing, and 83 received all three tests at both times. Control subjects took all three tests at the adult follow-up.

*Table 16-1: Handedness in Percent at Time of Referral and at Adult Age*

a) Handedness at Time of Referral Based on Grip Strength (I, in %)

| Group | Right | Ambilateral* | Left |
|-------|-------|--------------|------|
| 1 | 22.0 | 56.1 | 22.0 |
| 2 | 2.4 | 81.0 | 16.7 |
| 3 | 17.4 | 69.6 | 13.0 |

$n = 106$
chi square $= 8.98, p < .061$
* ambilaterality defined as + or – 1 $SD$ from mean of a control group

b) Handedness at Time of Referral Based on Grip Strength (II)
With a Rigid Definition of Ambilaterality

| Group | Right | Ambilateral** | Left |
|-------|-------|---------------|------|
| 1 | 58.5 | 14.6 | 26.8 |
| 2 | 54.8 | 21.4 | 23.8 |
| 3 | 69.6 | 8.7 | 21.7 |

$n = 106$
chi square $= 2.31, p < .68$
** Ambilaterality defined as r-l difference score $= 0$

### c) Handedness at Time of Referral Based on Questionnaire

| Group | Right | Ambilateral* | Left |
|---|---|---|---|
| 1 | 78.0 | 12.2 | 9.8 |
| 2 | 73.8 | 7.1 | 19.0 |
| 3 | 87.0 | 0.0 | 13.0 |
| 4** | 93.6 | 4.3 | 2.1 |

$n = 153$

chi square $= 11.38, p < .077$

\* ambilaterality defined as more than one and less than six activities with opposite hand or equally well with both hands.

\*\* Group 4 based on retrospective data, obtained at Phase II.

### d) Handedness at Adult Age Based on Questionnaire

| Group | Right | Ambilateral* | Left |
|---|---|---|---|
| 1 | 82.6 | 6.5 | 10.9 |
| 2 | 83.3 | 5.6 | 11.1 |
| 3 | 79.2 | 8.3 | 12.5 |
| 4 | 93.6 | 4.3 | 2.1 |

$n = 171$

chi square $= 4.36, p < .62$

\* ambilaterality defined as more than one and less than six activities performed with the opposite hand or equally well with both hands

### e) Handedness at Adult Age Based on Writing Time

| Group | Right | Left |
|---|---|---|
| 1 | 82.6 | 17.4 |
| 2 | 85.2 | 14.8 |
| 3 | 83.3 | 16.7 |
| 4 | 93.6 | 6.4 |

$n = 171$

chi square $= 2.92, p < .40$

The results indicate an increase of nondextrality in all three LD groups compared to controls (Table 16-1; Salter 1983; Salter & Spreen 1984). However, the hypothesis of increasing nondextrality as a function of degree of neuropathology (i.e., differences between groups 1 through 3) was not supported, either at time of referral or at the time of the Phase II recall. No 'dextral shift' over time was found, analyzing change scores based on self-report of handedness as well as on performance measures (writing time, grip strength). Hence, nondextrality cannot be viewed as a sign of a lag in maturation which eventually develops into dextrality during the teen years.

Two possible interpretations of these results can be made: (a) It is possible that the increased nondextrality in our sample was the result of selective referral, i.e., that nondextral children are more likely to be referred to our clinic if learning problems develop; (b) The alternate hypothesis, that LD subjects tend to have more pathological handedness, is more attractive. However, the failure to find differences between groups of definite, suggested, and no neurological deficit, suggests that, at least in our group, degree of neurological impairment is not a determining factor. It is more likely that LD children, even without neurological findings, have subtle dysfunctions which may trigger a change in handedness more often than in a nondisabled population. This is confirmed to some extent by the results reported in Section 13, which indicate that LD subjects without neurological findings at time of referral tend to have a surprisingly large number of soft neurological signs at adult age.

A subsidiary analysis contrasted younger (age 7:0 to 9:11) with older (age 10:0 to 13:11) subjects across the three referral age groups. No significant age contrast was found, suggesting that no significant shift in dextrality occurred at that age range.

In *summary*, we found an increased number of non-righthanded subjects in our sample of LD children. However, the notion that left-handedness or ambilaterality is increased in subjects with neurological findings was not supported. There was also no support for a 'shift' towards right-handedness over time: no significant change over 15 years was observed on several different measures of lateral preference.

## 17. Other Tests

Other tests administered during the Phase II recall included the Sentence Repetition Test and the Halstead Category Test (which had also been administered at time 1), the Bourdon Crossing-Out Test, Dichotic Listening, the Wechsler Memory Scale, the Controlled Word Association Test, the Purdue Pegboard Test, Finger Localization, and Right-Left Orientation. These tests were chosen because they tend to examine additional neuropsychological functions of interest and are relatively independent of intelligence and achievement tests.

The Halstead Category Test administered at referral age was either the children's version (age below 8) or the intermediate version (means 65.69, 55.43, and 59.75 errors, $p < .008$). During the Phase II recall, the adult version, Victoria revision (LaBreche 1982), was given. This revision, a reduced and restandardized version of the full-length Category Test, consists of four parts. The total error score and the error score for each part were examined for group differences. The scores for Part 1 did not reach significance, but the scores for parts 2 through 4 and the total error score did (Table 17-1).

*Table 17-1: Halstead Category Test Error Score (at age 25)*

| Group | 1 | 2 | 3 | Control | F | p< |
|---|---|---|---|---|---|---|
| Part 1 | 9.1 | 10.6 | 10.6 | 7.3 | 3.09 | .05 |
| Part 2 | 10.4 | 10.2 | 9.0 | 3.5 | 8.96 | .000 |
| Part 3 | 7.4 | 8.0 | 5.2 | 6.5 | 3.54 | .005 |
| Part 4 | 4.6 | 4.3 | 2.5 | 2.4 | 3.37 | .003 |
| Total Errors | 31.6 | 33.1 | 27.3 | 19.6 | 6.65 | .000 |
| SD | 14.7 | 14.0 | 13.0 | 12.7 | | |
| Total Errors for IQ-Matched Groups | 29.2 | 31.3 | 27.6 | 19.6 | 5.89 | .000 |

No significant sex differences were found. The intercorrelations between the Category Tests at referral age and during Phase II recall were strong and are described further in Section 25.

The Sentence Repetition Test (Spreen & Benton 1977) requires the immediate repetition of sentences of increasing length. The score reflects the number of syllables of the longest sentence correctly repeated. Significant group differences for this test existed at referral age (means 10.36, 11.25, and 11.86; $p < .013$). For the IQ-matched LD groups means at first testing were 11.19, 11.44, and 15.00 respectively. At the time of Phase II retest, a significant group difference of a linear type was found (12.8, 13.4, 14.0, and 15.5 for groups 1 to 4 respectively; $p < .01$). The significant difference was still present when groups were matched for IQ (13.74, 13.86, 14,08, 15.46 respectively, $F (3, 151) = 5.58$; $p < .001$). Correcting raw scores according to level of education did not improve group separation ($p < .001$, scores of 13.9, 14.7, 15.2, and 15.7 respectively).

The Bourdon Crossing-Out Test requires that the letters a, b and q (typed clearly at the top of the sheet) be crossed out in a page of randomly arranged letters, line by line. The test is considered a measure of concentration or focussed attention. Scores for this test, recently developed in our laboratory, consist of the number of lines completed after the first 2 and during the second 2 minutes. The mean scores for the four groups were 5.3, 5.7, 6.7, and 7.6 lines respectively for the first 2 minutes, and 5.0, 5.8, 6.7, and 7.2 lines for the second part. Both parts produced highly significant group differences ($p < .001$). Errors in crossing-out during the first and second half of this task were highest in group 3. The overall ANOVA was highly significant (.001), but group differences between the three LD groups were not significant. The same result was obtained after IQ matching (Table 17-2). These results are consistent with the findings of Herbst and Roesler (1986) who used serial addition (Dueker-Lienert Test) as a measure of concentration.

*Table 17-2: Bourdon Crossing Out Test at Adult Age with IQ Matched-Groups*

| Group | 1 | 2 | 3 | Control | $F$ | $p$ |
|---|---|---|---|---|---|---|
| Omission Errors | | | | | | |
| First Half | 11.83 | 8.62 | 12.42 | 6.18 | 4.81 | .003 |
| Second Half | 10.93 | 10.44 | 14.08 | 6.24 | 5.19 | .002 |

The dichotic listening test was administered to all subjects during the Phase II recall. The test consists of simultaneous presentation of two monosyllabic meaningful words, one to each ear. Eighteen trials of 3 word pairs each were given (four initial practice trials were not scored). The maximum possible raw score for either ear is 54. This test can be viewed as a test of immediate recall as well as a test of lateralization (ear preference).

In an analysis of ear preference, all 18 trials (six words each) were treated as individual experimental units (Clark & Spreen 1983) and scored as either right, left, or no preference. Hence, a perfectly right lateralized subject would be able to receive a score of 18. Table 17-3 shows the mean number of right-ear and left-ear preference trials for each group. A right-ear preference was found for all groups, but differences between the four groups were negligible. Right-ear preference was also not significantly different between IQ-matched groups. This result stands in contrast to the findings of Obrzut et al. (1985) who found a significantly weaker right-ear advantage in LD children. The total number of words repeated (regardless of ear of presentation) is also listed in Table 17-3. An increasingly better immediate recall score is found for groups 1, 2, and 3 respectively. This difference remained significant after IQ matching.

*Table 17-3: Dichotic Listening Performance and Ear Preference*

| Group | 1 | 2 | 3 | Control | $F$ | $p<$ |
|---|---|---|---|---|---|---|
| Total Words Correct | 41.86 | 44.08 | 47.28 | 50.04 | 7.18 | .001 |
| Total Words Correct | | | | | | |
| (IQ-matched LD grps) | 44.30 | 45.08 | 47.42 | 50.04 | 4.35 | .006 |
| Right Ear Preference | 9.00 | 9.76 | 10.21 | 9.47 | 0.60 | ns |
| Left Ear Preference | 4.44 | 4.64 | 4.17 | 4.38 | 0.19 | ns |
| No Ear Preference | 3.44 | 3.60 | 3.63 | 3.59 | 0.07 | ns |

A supplementary analysis of the dichotic listening data in relation to adult LD subtypes will be presented in conjunction with the subtype discussion in Section 21.

66

Another measure of short-term memory is the Wechsler Memory Test. All parts of this test were administered: memory passages (memory for stories), visual reproduction (memory for visual designs), paired associate learning, delayed memory for stories, digit span (see also WAIS-R, Section 16). The ANOVA between groups was significant for all of these subtests. Significant differences between individual group means (Student-Newman-Keuls procedure) were found for memory passages between groups 1 and 3, and 2 and 4, while the differences between groups 1 and 2, between 2 and 3, and between 3 and 4 were not significant. For visual reproduction, all differences except those between groups 2 and 3 were significant; for paired associates and for delayed memory and digit span, the three LD groups did not differ significantly from each other.

Table 17-5 : Wechsler Memory Scale Means for the Four Groups
(Group 1 to 3 Matched for IQ, Mean IQ — 97)

| Group Subtest | 1 | 2 | 3 | Control | F | p |
|---|---|---|---|---|---|---|
| Memory Passages | 72.9 | 74.4 | 90.0 | 99.5 | 4.04 | .008 |
| Visual Reproduction | 93.6 | 97.6 | 95.8 | 129.2 | 14.04 | .001 |
| Paired Associates | 149.5 | 149.0 | 150.8 | 182.7 | 11.69 | .001 |
| Delayed Memory | 44.8 | 47.6 | 50.2 | 72.8 | 6.52 | .001 |
| Digit Span | 8.0 | 8.0 | 7.8 | 10.7 | 14.26 | .001 |

As Table 17-5 shows, the ANOVA between groups after matching for IQ remains highly significant, but in the comparison between subgroups, differences between groups 1, 2, and 3 and between 3 and 4 for memory passages, between 1, 2, and 3 for visual reproduction and paired associates, delayed memory, and digit span do not reach significance. Hence, although a trend towards lower scores with the more neurologically impaired groups is noticed, only the difference between the three LD groups and the controls is significant after IQ matching.

Verbal fluency, first introduced by Thurstone (1938) as part of the Primary Mental Abilities Test, was measured with the Controlled Word Association Test (Spreen & Benton 1977). The subject is given 1 minute to find as many words as possible starting with a given letter. The procedure is used for each of three letters: F, A, and S.

The total number of words produced was significantly different for the four groups (.001). The differences between groups 1 and 2 and between groups 3 and 4 did not reach significance. A reanalysis with Groups 1 to 3 matched for IQ produced very similar results (Table 17-6). Applying corrections for grade level of education produced no change in these findings.

*Table 17-6: Mean Scores for Controlled Word Association*
*at Adult Age (Groups 1 to 3 Matched for IQ)*

| Group | 1 | 2 | 3 | Control |
|---|---|---|---|---|
| Raw Score | 31.66 | 31.52 | 39.29 | 43.12 |
| SD | 10.29 | 10.36 | 9.89 | 10.01 |

$F = 17.02; p < .001$

The Purdue Pegboard Test was given at the Phase II examination as a measure of finger dexterity and concentration. The test score consists of the number of pegs inserted correctly with the right hand, left hand, and using both hands. An 'assembly' score is produced by the number of correctly placed pegs with collars inserted separately, using both hands.

Differences between groups were highly significant for the right, left, both hands and for assembly. Group differences with IQ-matched samples also reached significance, except for the differences between groups 2 and 3 and between groups 3 and 4 (left-hand score), as well as between groups 2 and 3 for the other scores (Table 17-7).

*Table 17-7: Mean Purdue Pegboard Test Scores for the*
*Three LD Groups Matched for IQ and Controls*

| Group | 1 | 2 | 3 | Control | $F$ | $p <$ |
|---|---|---|---|---|---|---|
| *Pegboard Score* | | | | | | |
| Right Hand | 13.31 | 14.69 | 15.21 | 16.40 | 12.60 | .000 |
| Left Hand | 12.57 | 14.14 | 14.96 | 15.90 | 18.79 | .000 |
| Both Hands | 9.79 | 11.35 | 12.08 | 13.22 | 21.12 | .000 |
| Assembly | 29.34 | 33.83 | 36.09 | 41.68 | 21.47 | .000 |

It should be noted that, in spite of IQ matching, this test reflects significant differences in fine motor skills between groups with different degrees of neurological impairment. The results are consistent with Herbst and Roesler's (1986) findings on the Ozeretski test.

Finger Localization (Benton 1959) measures the ability to recognize the fingers touched on either hand, and to indicate which finger(s) it was by either naming or pointing to the picture of a hand. The differences between groups at Phase II were highly significant, even with IQ matched groups (Table 17-8).

Right-left orientation (Benton 1959) also showed highly significant differences between LD groups and controls, even with IQ-matching (Table 17-8). It should be noted that at the time of referral at age 10 the same test was given; the results, whether groups were matched for IQ or not, did not produce a significant difference at that time. At Phase II recall

*Table 17-8: Finger Localization and Right-Left Orientation*
*with LD Groups Matched for IQ*

| Group | 1 | 2 | 3 | Control | F | p |
|---|---|---|---|---|---|---|
| *Finger Localization* | | | | | | |
| Right Hand | 26.94 | 28.43 | 28.63 | 29.08 | 7.33 | .000 |
| Left Hand | 26.48 | 27.37 | 28.92 | 29.14 | 11.92 | .000 |
| *Right-Left Orientation* | | | | | | |
| Total Correct | 29.65 | 28.74 | 28.92 | 31.63 | 5.07 | .002 |
| Reversals | 1.97 | 1.94 | 1.92 | 2.00 | 1.33 | n.s. |
| Time (in seconds) | 173.58 | 182.73 | 165.00 | 151.28 | 6.31 | .000 |
| *At Referral Age* | | | | | | |
| Total Correct | 24.86 | 21.95 | 22.05 | | | |
| Reversals | 7.00 | 9.72 | 6.67 | | | |
| *Culver Hands and Feet Test* | | | | | | |
| Total Correct | 16.06 | 16.32 | 15.04 | 17.82 | 3.90 | .01 |
| Total Time | 89.00 | 89.68 | 74.83 | 60.31 | 6.33 | .000 |

the total correct score again did not differ significantly between the three LD groups after IQ matching, nor did the reversal score (number of consistent reversals of right and left) show significant group differences, even compared to the control group. It should be noted that reversals are typical for small children and are expected to disappear during maturation. The total time used for right-left orientation showed a significant ANOVA difference (.001), but separation between the three LD groups and between groups 3 and 4 was not significant before or after IQ matching.

An additional right-left orientation task with extended difficulty level, using pictures of hands and feet, was developed by Culver (1969). Part 1 of this test was administered during the Phase II examination. The ANOVA for the number of correct recognitions was significant (.01) both with and without IQ-matched groups. However, the differences between the three LD groups and (after IQ matching), between groups 1, 2, and 3 and between groups 1, 2, and 4 were not significant. Similarly, the time taken for this task showed significant differences overall, but not between the three LD groups or, after IQ matching, between groups 1, 2, and 4 (Table 17-8).

In *summary*, our LD subjects showed significantly more errors on all but the first part subscores as well as on the total score of the Halstead Category Test, both at referral and adult age. The Sentence Repetition Test indicated poorer short term memory at both times, increasing with degree of neurological impairment. Similar results were found for Word Fluency. At adult age, the Wechsler Memory Scale was poorer and the Bourdon crossing-out test indicated poorer concentration for all LD groups. Similar findings were obtained for finger dexterity (Purdue Pegboard Test), finger localization, and right-left orientation. Dichotic listening at adult age also showed better word recall for controls and neurologically unimpaired subjects, but right-ear preference was common to all subjects and did not differ between groups.

## c. Personality and Psychiatric Problems

Social maladjustment and emotional problems have frequently been noticed more often in LD children and adolescents than in the general population of the same age. As an example, a recent book by Chapman and Boersma (1980) studied in detail the affective characteristics of LD children and noted in particular a 'relative negative academic self-concept, reflecting low self-perception of abilities', external locus of control, and poor self-perception along with negative school attitude, and diminishing levels of self-confidence; this was evident both in self-perception and in the perception of parents and teachers.

One common viewpoint suggests that emotional problems are more likely to develop because of continuous failure experiences in school, parental pressure, frustration, and rejection, i.e. they represent a secondary reaction to LD (Wender 1971; Denhoff 1973). However, it has also been argued that the LD itself is the result of certain personality traits or emotional problems which affect attending behaviour and learning. Finally, recent authors have adopted the position that both LD and emotional problems have their origin in a common third factor, variously described as cerebral dysfunction, maturational disorder, or central processing deficit (Willerman 1973, Wolff & Hurwitz 1973).

Rourke and Fisk (1981) have adopted the latter view, and present a survey of some pertinent studies. Using the Personality Inventory for Children, Porter and Rourke (1985) found that, in 100 children with learning or perceptual problems, means on scales measuring personality functioning remained in the average range, while the academic and intellectual screening scales were significantly elevated (reflecting the referral problem of these children). However, a Q-factor analysis of the data revealed that 75% of the children could be separated into specific subtypes: The largest subtype (46% = 37 subjects) showed minimal scale variations and no significant scale elevations; the second subtype ($n$=20) was seriously disturbed, tentatively labelled as childhood depression, poor interpersonal functioning, social isolation, and poor self-esteem; a third subtype ($n$=10) expressed primarily 'somatic concerns', including a high number of visual problems; the fourth subtype ($n$=13) was described as overactive, restless, distractible, showing poor ability to maintain concentration and attention ('hyperactive'). A replication study (Fisk & Rourke 1984) confirmed these findings : 70% of this population could be classified into the first three subtypes (representing 50, 25 and 25% of the classified population), but subtype 4 could not be replicated. Within subtype 2 and 3 the degree of psychopathology was greater; in these subtypes the VIQ was greater than the PIQ by 10 points or more.

Ozols and Rourke (1985) also attempted to relate two groups differing in measures of social sensitivity to subtypes of achievement and intellectual and neuropsychological disabilities. The results were tentative and suggested that, at age 8 to 11, children with poor auditory-verbal and language-related abilities differed from children with poor visual-spatial abilities on tasks requiring the description of feelings expressed in pictures and in making inferences from pictures showing social situations. A study by Strang (1981) showed that 8- to 11-year-old children with markedly different patterns of linguistic and visuo-spatial abilities differed in patterns of personality functioning as well. Strang's study also seemed to indicate that older LD children did not show more emotional maladaptation than younger LD children. This last finding would seem to run contrary to the notion that continuing failure experience builds up to more and more severe emotional problems in the growing child.

No previous research has directly addressed the long-term development and the adult occurrence rate of emotional problems in LD. A follow-up by Bruck (1985) seems to suggest an increased degree of maladjustment in the late teen age range, but no childhood measures are available to indicate the developmental progression. The current study also has no direct measures of the emotional status in childhood, although a retrospective exploration of that topic was attempted in both the parent and student interview at Phase I. Direct measures of personality adjustment as well as standardized interview items pertaining to the emotional adjustment as late teenagers and as adults were included in Phase I and II of the project. The following section will review some of these findings.

A description of the personal characteristics of our participants can be obtained from several sources: (a) at age 19 (Phase I follow-up) each participant filled in an adjustment inventory (Bell 1962), (b) at the same time, parents filled in a rating scale describing personality characteristics of their child, (c) the interviewers filled in an interviewer rating scale about the behaviour during the interview, (d) at age 25 (Phase II follow-up) the full MMPI was administered (see section 19), (e) interviewer and examiner filled in a rating scale describing the behaviour during that period, (f) finally, subjects were asked a number of direct questions about themselves pertaining to personal characteristics, either requiring their own judgement ('are you satisfied with your life now?') or asking for information ('have you ever been described as hyperactive?').

71

## 18. Self-Descriptions, Ratings, and Behaviour
   During the Interviews and Tests

During the Phase I interview, a tendency towards doubting their own judgement was found most frequently in Group 1. Asked whether they were generally satisfied with their life, there was also a trend towards more negative responses in Groups 1 and 2, the two brain-dysfunction groups. A significant difference between groups was found on the question whether subjects saw themselves as different from others - with a linear trend from group 1 to 4 (57.4, 49.2, 37.0, and 31.4% respectively; $p < .04$). This question was repeated during the Phase II interview. The trend of responses remained significant (75.0, 71.0, 46.2, and 37.0% respectively; $p < .01$).

Immediately after the Phase II recall, each subject was rated according to the behaviour during the interview and during the testing (Appendix 3). The 5-point scales usually ranged from the most marked positive expression of a trait (e.g., 'unusually determined to be right, competitive, fearful of failure') to the negative extreme (e.g.,'careless, inattentive, little effort'). Seven scales were rated by the interviewer, nine by the test examiner (who was not aware of group membership), and five scales by both. These latter scales included grooming, maturity of behaviour, body type, whether the interview and test results could be considered as valid, and whether a follow-up interview by the principal investigator would be indicated. The other scales ranged from the degree of manifest anxiety exhibited to how well rapport was established. Interviewer and test examiner's ratings correlated moderately and positively (anxiety $r = .53$; verbal output .71; manner of relating to the examiner .53; appropriateness of behaviour .47; motivation .52; self-confidence .56; rapport with examiner .30). These correlations probably do not reflect merely the reliability of the rating, but also true differences of behaviour depending on whether an interview was conducted or whether the participant was asked to do his best on the tests administered.

The 12 rating scales were submitted to a principal component factor analysis which also included the sum of the 12 ratings as well as age and IQ at referral age. Six factors were found: The first factor had loadings primarily on grooming, ability to concentrate, and motivation; the second consisted mainly of 'appropriateness of behaviour', factor 3 was a combination of ratings on 'grooming' and body type; factor 4 referred to verbal output and manner of relating to the examiner; factor 5 showed residual loadings of IQ and recommendations for follow-up counselling; factor 6 was an age-related residual factor.

This analysis shows that no 'general' factor accounts for most of the rating results, and therefore presents indirect evidence that the ratings were done individually, and do not suffer from a general 'halo-effect'.

No group differences were found on grooming, but females were significantly more often described as neat, and males more often as 'sloppy, careless'.

The four groups differed significantly on verbal output during the interview: Groups 3 and 4 (mean ratings: 3.44 and 3.36) were more loquacious, while more subjects in groups 1 and 2 were described as 'taciturn, no spontaneous conversation' or as 'quiet' (mean ratings 3.01 and 3.03; $p < .05$). A nonsignificant age trend was also noted: older subjects were rated as more verbal than were younger ones ($p < .09$).

The groups also differed significantly on the ratings of appropriateness of behaviour. Combining the ratings of interviewer and examiner, control group subjects were described as more appropriate (mean 2.88) than the three LD groups (means 3.11, 3.00, 3.14, $p < .01$). Ratings of maturity of behaviour were significantly different between groups. The control group was more often rated as serious, while the LD groups were rated as average, and an 'impulsive' rating was found most often in the two brain-damaged groups (means: 3.07, 3.01, 2.96 for groups 1, 2 and 3, and 2.72 for controls; $p < .01$). A significant sex difference was also found with the females more often described as serious and the males more often as impulsive.

Rating of self-confidence only differed between sexes, but not by group: males were more often in the middle range of ratings, while females were found more often in the extreme groups (overly self-critical, or overly confident and bragging).

Rapport was better established during the interview with subjects in groups 3 and 4 (mean ratings: 4.92 and 4.92 vs. 4.61 and 4.76 in groups 1 and 2; $p < .01$). Females in general showed better motivation, but groups also differed significantly on this rating with poorer motivation found in groups 1 and 2 (means 2.88, 2.80 and 2.66 for groups 1, 2 and 3; 2.57 for controls, $p < .04$). An age effect was observed: older subjects appeared somewhat better motivated than younger ones ($p < .11$).

In an attempt to summarize the information on several rating scales, the number of times a person was rated as '1', '2', '3', etc. on all scales was counted. The only significant group difference was on the number of '2' ratings, which reflects a moderately negative rating ('3' = average). Group 1 subjects had more of these ratings than group 2 and 3, while group 4 had the lowest number of such ratings.

In addition to the ratings of behaviour and appearance during the interview, an attempt was made to describe special characteristics of each participant in 'vignette' form, i.e., in a narrative description approximately half a page in length. By their very nature, such vignettes are not suitable for statistical evaluation. Sorting procedures were used to evaluate the vignettes more formally, but they served mainly as descriptive information for characteristics which are not readily codable (for example one vignette describes a participant who refused any appointment before 1 pm because

73

he slept until noon, though unemployed; he then broke four appointments, and could only be persuaded to come by the promise of 'payment' for his time).

In *summary*, LD subjects at age 18 tended to doubt their own judgement and saw themselves as different more often than controls. Ratings of appropriateness and maturity of behaviour were better for group 3 subjects and controls than for groups 1 and 2. The latter two groups also had more difficulty in establishing rapport during the interview.

### 19. Emotional Adjustment as Measured with Personality Inventories

While other questions and rating scales pertaining to personal adjustment have already been described earlier (Section 18), two formal measures of adjustment were used in this study: (a) the Bell Adjustment Inventory was administered at the Phase I follow-up (Peter & Spreen 1979), and (b) the Minnesota Multiphasic Personality Inventory was administered at the Phase II follow-up. Both are questionnaire tests, requiring the individual to answer yes or no to a number of printed statements. The purpose was to obtain more standardized measures about the psychiatric and emotional adjustment of our subjects as adults . Other studies have described LD subjects as more prone to emotional and psychiatric problems later in life, but such descriptions have not always been consistent; some investigators have claimed that the child 'outgrows' most of the adverse affective concomitants associated with LD.

*Bell Inventory and Parent Rating Scale at Age 18*

The Bell Personal Adjustment Inventory was shortened from the original 200-item form by eliminating the items of the masculinity/femininity and the hostility scale. The remaining 140 items produced scores on four scales, home adjustment, health adjustment, social adjustment, and emotional adjustment. Split-half reliability was satisfactory; the four scales showed Spearman-Brown coefficients between .83 and .88.

Combining the three LD groups, a significant difference between LD and control subjects was found for all four scales: Home, health, social and emotional adjustment (Table 19-1).

*Table 19-1: Bell Adjustment Inventory Scores at Phase I*

| Scale | Group | 1 | 2 | 3 | Control | $p <$ | males | females | $p <$ |
|---|---|---|---|---|---|---|---|---|---|
| Home Adjustment | | 11.45 | 13.69 | 10.02 | 7.23 | .05 | 10.06 | 12.38 | .02 |
| Health Adjustment | | 10.12 | 10.58 | 8.23 | 6.28 | .05 | 8.12 | 10.63 | .004 |
| Social Adjustment | | 16.33 | 16.45 | 16.96 | 13.55 | .05 | 14.79 | 17.69 | .004 |
| Emotional Adjustment | | 12.56 | 12.95 | 12.39 | 8.53 | .05 | 10.24 | 14.34 | .001 |

A multivariate analysis, using the four Bell scales as dependent variables, indicated that presence of a learning disability was a significant predictor of poor adjustment ($p < .001$) for all scales and for each scale individually, accounting for 22.79% of the variance; sex was also a significant predictor (15.92%); intelligence contributed 5.48, age 5.62% of the variance.

A behaviour rating scale (based on Hanvik et al. 1961) designed to identify behaviour typically associated with cerebral dysfunction was given to the parents during the Phase I follow-up where it was completed under the supervision of the interviewer. The interviewer clarified any ambiguities, and stressed the need to rate current behaviour of their son or daughter. The 30 6-point scores were reduced by factor analysis to six composite scores: (1) antisocial-acting out, (2) disorganized, incautious, careless, forgetful, (3) emotionally dependent, (4) insecure, sensitive, fearful, (5) inactive, clumsy and uncoordinated, unsociable, (6) tense, anxious, insomniac. The factor analysis was conducted with all 244 participating parents of Phase I and repeated with exlusion of all subjects with IQs of less than 70 and including 28 additional subjects; the second analysis replicated essentially the same results.

The four groups were compared on the six composite scores. The multivariate test was significant; three composite scores provided significant contrast between groups (Table 19-2). The pattern consistently associated with the brain-damaged group included emotionally dependent, clumsy/inactive/unsociable behaviour; the group with minimal neurological signs was described by parents more often as disorganized/incautious and sensitive/jealous/insecure; the three LD groups differed from controls significantly on variables which described disorganized/incautious and inactive/unsociable as well as antisocial/acting-out behaviour.

Table 19-2: Six Composite Behaviours Based on Parent Rating at Age 19

| Group<br>Behaviour | 1 | 2 | 3 | 4 | $p<$ |
|---|---|---|---|---|---|
| antisocial | 2.94 | 2.96 | 2.96 | 2.40 | .148 |
| disorganized | 2.98 | 3.18 | 2.66 | 2.41 | .001 |
| emotionally dependent | 3.79 | 3.49 | 3.29 | 3.10 | .001 |
| sensitive/insecure | 3.11 | 3.30 | 2.93 | 2.91 | .172 |
| inactive/unsociable | 3.50 | 3.18 | 2.77 | 2.49 | .001 |
| tense/insomniac | 2.17 | 2.88 | 2.69 | 2.27 | .724 |

Manova: $F=13.008$, $df=6$, $p < .001$, % variance=25.6

The multivariate analyses did not show significant interaction effects, but there were significant effects of sex ($p < .001$), and IQ level ($p < .001$). Females appeared to have more deviant outcome scores than males, and the brighter subjects achieved better adjustment than those at lower IQ levels. IQ level affected significantly the outcome on four variables (emotionally dependent, insecure/sentive, inactive/unsociable, tense).

*MMPI at Age 25*

Because of time constraints during the Phase II testing, the MMPI was usually begun under supervision at the laboratory, but often completed at home and mailed back. Because of poor reading skills, the taped version was given in a few instances and for a few other participants the test had to be abandoned. Failure to return the questionnaire accounted for additional subject loss (see Table 1-2). Finally, a few records were excluded because of abnormal validity scales in conjunction with poor reading level. The records of 153 subjects, 43 subjects in Group 1, 47 in Group 2, 17 in Group 3, and 46 in Group 4, were available for analysis. After an analysis of MMPI profiles for good and poor readers, the analysis was further restricted to participants who obtained a reading comprehension level (PIAT) of at least grade 7 (Burnside 1986). This reduced the available MMPI protocols to 128. All MMPI analyses using T-scores were based on the age-appropriate Colligan norms (Colligan et al. 1983).

Group differences for the 3 validity, the 10 clinical scales, and 7 selected special or subscales were examined (Burnside 1986; Rusell 1984; Russell & Spreen 1984). The special scales included Subjective Depression (D1), Mental Dullness (D4), Brooding (D5), Denial of Social Anxiety (Hyl), Social Alienation (Pd4A), Lack of Ego Mastery (Sc2B), and Ego strength (Es). The first six of the subscales were constructed from the clinical scales by Harris and Lingoes (1955, 1968) reflecting mainly unhappiness, lack of self-confidence, feelings of inferiority, brooding, and social alienation. Ego

Table 19-3: Univariate F-Tests between groups on MMPI Scales

| Scale | $F(1, 127)$ | $p <$ |
|---|---|---|
| L ('lie scale') | 6.06 | .011 |
| F (validity scale) | 15.44 | .001 |
| K (correction scale) | 4.42 | .038 |
| 1 'Hypochondriasis' | .69 | n.s. |
| 2 'Depression' | 2.96 | .088 |
| 3 'Hysteria' | .14 | n.s. |
| 4 'Psychopathic Deviate' | 8.41 | .004 |
| 5 'Masculinity/Femininity' | .37 | n.s. |
| 6 'Paranoia' | 6.59 | .011 |
| 7 'Psychasthenia' | 3.72 | .056 |
| 8 'Schizophrenia' | 5.67 | .019 |
| 9 'Mania' | .65 | n.s. |
| 0 'Social Introversion' | 3.89 | .051 |

strength (Barron 1953) has been shown to reflect good adjustment; high scorers are unlikely to have motionla problems.

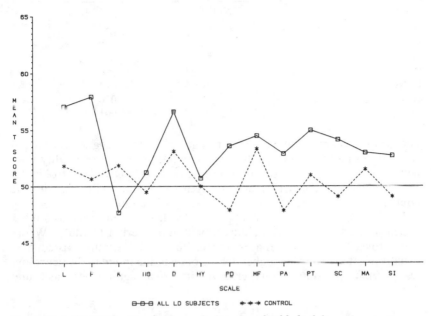

*Figure 19-1: MMPI-Profiles for formerly learning-disabled adults and controls*

A MANOVA of the three validity and 10 clinical scales produced a significant group separation ($p < .001$). Examination of the univariate $F$ tests for each of the scales showed significance for all scales except Hy, Hs, Mf, and Ma (Table 19-3, Figure 19-1). Group comparisons showed only minor significant differences between LD groups, so that only the main contrast between all LD subjects and controls can be interpreted with confidence (Figure 19-1). In all scales except K, the LD subjects showed higher scores than controls, indicating increased tendencies in the direction of depression, acting-out tendencies, social sensitivity, obsessions, compulsions or phobias, bizarre experiences or thoughts, and social withdrawal or shyness. The lower K-scale scores are usually found in people with social distress and with poor self-concept.

The analysis of the subscale scores also showed significant group separation ($p < .007$) for the combined LD groups compared to controls (Table 19-4, Figure 19-2). Multivariate differences obtained for both male and female participants. However, LD women showed more disturbed scores on 6 subscales (subjective depression, mental dullness, brooding, social alienation, lack of ego mastery), but lower scores on the scale measuring

77

| Scale | $F(1, 127)$ | $p<$ |
|---|---|---|
| D1 | 7.45 | .007 |
| D4 | 7.53 | .007 |
| D5 | 6.93 | .010 |
| Hy1 | .11 | n.s. |
| Pd4A | 6.36 | .013 |
| Sc2B | 5.94 | .016 |
| Es | 20.27 | .001 |

denial of social anxiety and the ego-strength scale. This suggests poorer ego strength and a tendency to admit to social anxieties more readily than control women. The significant difference between LD and control males was produced by two scales, ego strength and mental dullness, with the control group showing scores in the 'healthy' direction.

In general, the results lend support to evidence from previous studies which showed a pattern of maladjustment in formerly LD adults. Where trends towards group differences among the three LD groups existed, they usually pointed towards a higher degree of maladjustment in the neurologically impaired groups. However, since statistical significance was found

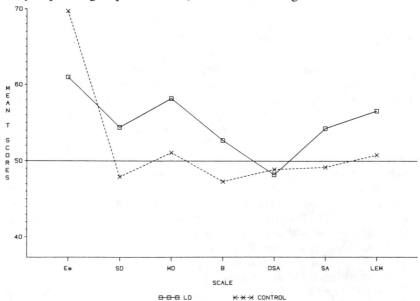

Figure 19-2: MMPI subscales and research scales for formerly learning-disabled adults and controls.

for only a few of these differences, this trend should be treated with caution.

Burnside (1986) also analyzed factor scores derived from the MMPI by Tryon, Stein, and Chu (Stein 1968). Again, the differences between the three LD groups did not reach multivariate significance, but the LD groups compared to controls showed a significant difference ($F = 3.20, p = .004$), based on 5 of the seven factors (Body Symptoms, Suspicion, Depression, Autism and Disruptive Thought, Tension and Worry). In addition, Taylor's (1953) manifest anxiety scale showed a significantly lower score for control women, while LD men and women scored higher than control men. This result seems to confirm the low denial of social anxiety found earlier for control women. Finally, the alcoholism scale (McAndrew 1965) showed a significant group effect ($F [3,125] = 2.57, p = .057$) with the highest score found in group 3 men.

The means for the individual groups rarely exceeded the traditional cut-off point for psychopathology, i.e., a standard score of 70. Scores in that range would be expected in only 2.3% of the population based on the normal distribution curve. Colligan et al. (1983) found such elevations in 1.9 to 3.1% of their normative sample. In our LD population the frequency of high $T$-scores frequently exceeded these expectations. A more detailed analysis of 'high-scorers' ($T$ values over 70) showed that these were least frequent in the control group with increased frequencies for scale 2 and 7 in group 2 and for scale 9 in group 3. 'High-scorers' on the subscales again were least frequent in the control group (Table 19-5). While no statistical

Table 19-5: Pe͞    ͤͨ of MMPI-Scores in the Disturbed Range (T-score > 70) by Group

| Group | 1 | 2 | 3 | 4 |
|-------|----|----|----|----|
| n | 30 | 38 | 15 | 46 |
| *Scale* | | | | |
| L | 17 | 11 | 0 | 15 |
| F | 13 | 13 | 13 | 2 |
| K | 3 | 5 | 7 | 0 |
| l(Hs) | 7 | 11 | 7 | 0 |
| 2(D) | 10 | 13 | 7 | 4 |
| 3(Hy) | 3 | 5 | 7 | 4 |
| 4(Pd) | 7 | 11 | 7 | 2 |
| 5(Mf) | 7 | 11 | 0 | 4 |
| 6(Pa) | 3 | 5 | 7 | 2 |
| 7(Pt) | 7 | 13 | 7 | 7 |
| 8(Sc) | 10 | 8 | 7 | 0 |
| 9(Ma) | 3 | 3 | 13 | 4 |
| 0(Si) | 3 | 5 | 0 | 0 |

comparisons could be performed with the relatively low number of high-scorers, the trend is fairly clear. Comparison by sex also indicated, that, except for the depression scales, high-scorers tended to be more often male than female.

Only three subjects showed the classical three-scale elevation described as the 'neurotic triad', and three subjects showed the hyperactivity/sociopathy elevation (scales 4, 8, 9); all six subjects belonged to group 3.

In *summary*, the Bell Adjustment Inventory at age 18 showed that the LD population had significantly poorer home, health, social, and emotional adjustment. The behaviour rating scales given at the same age suggested that our group 1 subjects were more emotionally dependent and showed more clumsy, inactive, and unsociable behaviour. Group 2 was more often described as disorganized, incautious, and sensitive, jealous, and insecure. At age 25, the MMPI confirmed poor emotional adjustment on most of the clinical scales, subscales, and research scales. For this population, the picture of lack of self-confidence, brooding, depression, emerges, especially for females, while males more often showed tendencies towards autistic behaviour and disruptive thought.

# d. Multivariate Analysis of Groups of Variables and Prediction

### 20. Predicting Adjustment and Group Membership on the Basis of the Initial Test Results and Socio-Economic Status

These investigations (Spreen & Lawriw 1980; Spreen 1984) addressed two questions: (a) The concurrent validity of the tests obtained at the time of the original referral in discriminating the three groups of LD children, formed on the basis of their neurological examination; (b) the predictive validity of these tests in regard to outcome at age 19 (Phase I), i.e., in terms of later emotional, social, occupational, and health adjustment. Such predictive validity has, of course, not been seriously claimed for neuropsychological tests nor is it an essential part of the validation procedure for such tests. Numerous intervening variables, such as treatment, education, employment opportunities, and occupational training may confound the long-term predictive validity of any test, even if we disregard the influence of personality variables. However, since cognitive tests of the IQ variety are usually assumed to have some predictive validity, at least for educational progress and achievement, the working hypothesis was adopted that tests given at age 10 may show some predictive validity for educational and other long-term adjustment.

Most studies of concurrent validity are limited to correlational validity with other tests or with academic achievement, especially for the WISC (Matarazzo 1972). In addition, IQ tests have been demonstrated to have concurrent validity for adaptive behaviour in terms of school grades (Conry & Plant 1965), with occupational attainment, income, socio-economic status and various physical characteristics; correlation coefficients range from .20 for job success to .70 for educational attainment and .90 for mental retardation. Studies of true predictive validity over longer periods of time are usually concerned with prediction of achievement during the elementary school years (Satz, Taylor, Friel & Fletcher 1978); studies with tests predicting adult adjustment are virtually absent. Werner and Smith (1977) come closest to this question, using a Cattell IQ, congenital defect indicators, activity level and various environmental and parental indicators at age 2, combined with pediatric assessment, a Primary Mental Abilities test and various other measures at age 10 in predicting problems during puberty in a longitudinal design. It should be noted that none of their predictors exceeded an $r$ of .24 (except for an r of .38 for the Cattell IQ at age 2 for girls), and that the multiple $r$ for boys was only .37, for girls .35, based only son the age-2 data; inclusion of the age-10 data did not improve the predictive validity. One reason for the relatively low predictive validity in this study may be the nature of most adjustment data (interview results); correlations between rating scales and 'real life' (interview) data tend to become somewhat spurious because of a variety of measurement problems as well as because of differences in actual content area (Cattell 1978; Nesselroade & Delhees 1966).

In the current study, 51 test or subtest scores obtained at age 10 were treated as predictor variables. These scores were reduced to 40 on the basis of: availability of a given score for the majority of our subjects, sufficient frequency of occurrence of a given score, lack of high correlation with other test variables, and meaningfulness in the context of an exploratory factor analysis of all test scores. From the 219 bits of information gathered at Phase I of the current study, 50 were selected according to the following criteria: significance of between-groups analysis of variance (or chi-square where appropriate), exclusion of highly correlated variables, variance accounted for in a multiple stepwise regression analysis in relation to the original test variables, and meaningfulness of the variable in the context of an exploratory factor analysis of all variables belonging to a given area (e.g., all variables relating to health adjustment).

*Analysis 1: Discrimination of groups on the basis of predictor and outcome variables.*

A preliminary question, namely the discrimination between the three LD groups based on the test data obtained at the time of referral, was asked first. A positive answer to this question would strengthen the expectation of good predictive validity over time; on the other hand, if group discrimination is weak, long-term predictive validity would appear to be questionable.

The test data obtained at the time of referral were used in a discriminant function analysis. As Table 20-1 shows, these data discriminated significantly between LD groups with definite, minimal, and no neurological findings at the time of referral. The overall correct classification rate is almost 71%. The table also lists the variables contributing to the discriminant function.

*Table 20-1: Discriminant Function between 8- to 12-Year Old*
*LD Subjects with Definite, Minimal, and no Neurological Findings on Test*
*Variables, and List of Best Predictor Variables*

| Actual Group | Predicted Group Membership | | | |
| | 1 | 2 | 3 | *n* |
| --- | --- | --- | --- | --- |
| 1 Definite | 73.1 | 23.1 | 3.8 | 52 |
| 2 Minimal | 14.5 | 65.2 | 20.3 | 69 |
| 3 No neurological findings | 8.8 | 11.8 | 79.4 | 34 |

Overall Correct Prediction: 70.9%.

Best Predictors:

| Step Entered | Variable | *F* | *p* < |
| --- | --- | --- | --- |
| 1 | WISC Coding | 15.43 | .001 |
| 2 | WISC Similarities | 12.38 | .001 |
| 3 | Embedded Figures, Correct | 12.00 | .001 |
| 4 | WISC Picture Arrangement | 10.85 | .001 |
| 5 | Sentence Repetition | 7.97 | .001 |
| 6 | Full Scale IQ (WISC) | 7.52 | .001 |
| 7 | WISC Vocabulary | 6.73 | .001 |
| 8 | Hand Grip Strength | 5.29 | .006 |
| 9 | Benton Vis.Retention Test, Errors | 4.82 | .01 |
| 10 | WISC Arithmetic | 4.76 | .01 |
| 11 | Embedded Figures, Overtime | 4.42 | .01 |
| 12 | Benton VRT, Displacements | 3.67 | .03 |
| 13 | Writing Name, right hand | 2.98 | .05 |
| 14 | Trail Making Test | 2.83 | .06 |
| 15 | WISC Information | 2.74 | .06 |

The test variables at time of referral (predictor variables) were submitted to a principal component analysis (varimax rotation) in order to obtain an estimate of cohesion for future analysis of their relationship to outcome variables. Table 20-2 shows the factors obtained. Of the eight factors with eigenvalues greater than 1, the first appears to be a general intelligence/ school achievement factor, the second a visuo-motor factor. Factors 3 to 8 are relatively specific (residual), covering writing, specific errors on the Visual Retention Test, lateral dominance, embedded figures and sex of subject. Oblique rotation obtained an optimal fit at a delta of .30 (with Kaiser normalization). The factors remained essentially unchanged with only one correlation (between factors 1 and 4) at a level of .43; the remaining between-factor correlations were at .27 or less, suggesting a fair degree of independence of the contribution of each of the eight factors.

*Table 20-2: Principal Component Factors of Tests Variables at Time of Referral*

| Factor | Description of Scores | Eigenvalue | Cumulative Proportion of Total Variance |
|---|---|---|---|
| 1 | Full Scale IQ, vocabulary, information comprehension, similarities, sentence repetition | 7.36 | .27 |
| 2 | BVRT errors, distortions, substitutions, Embedded Figures correct | 2.15 | .35 |
| 3 | Writing, right hand, Trail Making, Coding BVRT perseverations | 1.72 | .42 |
| 4 | Lateral Dominance, Handedness | 1.23 | .56 |
| 5 | BVRT misplacements, omissions, Grip Strength | 1.47 | .47 |
| 6 | Sex of S, Coding, Grip Strength | 1.31 | .52 |
| 7 | BVRT perseverations, rotations | 1.16 | .61 |
| 8 | Embedded Figures, correct in overtime, Sentence Repetition | 1.07 | .65 |

*Analysis 2: Discrimination of Groups Based on Outcome Variables.*

A further preliminary analysis involved an investigation of the discrimination between groups at the time of Phase I follow-up in order (1) to review the relative contribution of each outcome variable to discrimination, (2) to find meaningful groupings of outcome variables, and (3) to eliminate redundancies, in preparation for relating these variables to the test predictor variables described above. Table 20-3 shows the discriminant function between the four groups (including the control group) and the outcome variables contributing at a $p < .01$ or better to the discriminant function analysis.

*Table 20-3: Four-Group Discriminant Function of Long-Term Outcome Variables between LD Groups with Definite, Minimal and No Neurological Findings at Time of Referral and Controls*

| | | Predicted Group Membership | | | | |
|---|---|---|---|---|---|---|
| Actual Group | | 1 | 2 | 3 | 4 | *n* |
| 1 | Definite neurological findings | 71.2 | 13.5 | 13.5 | 1.9 | 52 |
| 2 | Minimal neurological findings | 15.9 | 66.7 | 11.6 | 5.8 | 69 |
| 3 | No neurological findings | 2.9 | 14.7 | 76.5 | 5.9 | 34 |
| 4 | Control | 1.9 | 5.8 | 1.9 | 90.4 | 52 |

Overall Correct Classification: 75.36 %
(Classification Rate when all 51 variables are forced: 78.7%)

Best Contributing Outcome Variables to 4-Group Discriminant Function

| Step entered | Variable/Question | Wilk's lambda | *F* |
|---|---|---|---|
| 1 | Previous learning disability | .744 | 23.17** |
| 2 | Difficulty finding a job | .635 | 17.14 |
| 3 | Contacted hearing/eye specialist | .559 | 14.69 |
| 4 | Passed last grade attended in school | .501 | 13.18 |
| 5 | Age when S took first job | .456 | 12.07 |
| 6 | Home adjustment (Bell Inventory) | .428 | 10.89 |
| 7 | Rated manner of relating to interviewer | .400 | 10.13* |
| 8 | Follow-up/treatment recommended by interviewer | .376 | 9.50 |
| 9 | Parent rating: Destructiveness & Assentmindedness | .356 | 8.97 |
| 10 | Have you ever dated? | .338 | 8.50 |
| 11 | Sees father fairly often | .321 | 8.13 |
| 12 | Attended college | .307 | 7.74 |
| 13 | Is frequently phoned by friends | .296 | 7.39 |
| 14 | Emotional adjustment (Inventory) | .284 | 7.09 |
| 15 | Submissiveness (Inventory) | .274 | 6.83 |
| 16 | Number of accidents | .264 | 6.58 |
| 17 | Type of present job | .257 | 6.33 |
| 18 | Total number of jobs held | .249 | 6.11 |
| 19 | Does family get along together? | .242 | 5.91 |
| 20 | Do you get along with classmates? | .235 | 5.71 |
| 21 | Contacted psychiatrist/psychologist | .230 | 5.53 |
| 22 | Age when entered preschool | .223 | 5.38 |
| 23 | Involvement in school activities | .218 | 5.22 |
| 24 | Held office in school or club | .213 | 5.08 |
| 25 | Are you working now? | .207 | 4.95 |
| 26 | Does your present job require the best of your abilities? | .293 | 4.82 |

| 27 | Health problem before the original referral | .199 | 4.69 |
| 28 | Number of sisters | .194 | 4.59 |
| 29 | Have you come to the attention of the police? | .189 | 4.48 |
| 30 | Is often visited by friends | .186 | 4.38 |
| 31 | Likes to give and seek affection (Parent rating) | .181 | 4.29 |
| 32 | Has contacted a physician | .177 | 4.20 |
| 33 | Has concern for feelings of others (Parent rating) | .174 | 4.11 |
| 34 | Health adjustment | .171 | 4.01 |

** first six variables significant at $p < .0001$
* variable 7 and below significant at $p < .01$

While variable 1 and 4 may seem redundant in that they deal with the observation of the participant that an LD existed, it should be stressed that these variables contributed to a 4-group discriminant function, i.e.,to the differentiation of the three LD groups from each other as well as from control subjects. As expected from Table 20-2, contrasting all three LD groups jointly with the control group in a 2-group discriminant function analysis, yields an extremely high significant discrimination rate (95.17%).

*Analysis 3: Prediction of outcome areas from referral test variables.*

We can now proceed to the question of predictive validity. A first analysis searched for the relationship of each test variable with each of seven outcome areas: School experience, job and employment, learning and health problems, treatment, social adjustment, personal experience, family and family relation. A stepwise regression analysis for each test for each of these outcome areas is summarized in Table 20-4. Each value represents a multiple $R$-square of the test in relation to the group of variables representing the outcome area.

As expected, some of the more specialized tests, e.g., sound recognition, right- and left-handed writing time, made only a minimal contribution to the regression in most areas. On the other hand, some basic achievement test scores, class grade attended at the time of referral, and grip strength, contributed consistently, though not always highly, to most outcome areas. The relatively spotty contribution of IQ subtests and the contribution of IQ-scores themselves to only four outcome areas is surprising.

To investigate the relationship between several predictors and several outcome variables, the canonical analysis is an appropriate tool of analysis. In this case, representative factor-weighted scores at the time of referral

Table 20-4: Contribution of Individual Test Variables to
Prediction of Clusters of Outcome Variables

| Test Score | Areas of Outcome | | | | | | |
|---|---|---|---|---|---|---|---|
| | 1 | 2 | 3 | 4 | 5 | 6 | 7 |
| WRAT Coding | 67 | 58 | 57 | 53 | 66 | 47 | 54 |
| WRAT Spelling | 57 | 42 | 42 | 29 | 51 | 31 | 36 |
| WRAT Arithmetic | 52 | 38 | 49 | 38 | 47 | 51 | 34 |
| WRAT Reading | 43 | 28 | 27 | 23 | 38 | 28 | 28 |
| Class Grade | 44 | 30 | 41 | 29 | 42 | 44 | 30 |
| WISC Information | 35 | 31 | | | 35 | | |
| WISC Digit Span | 34 | | 26 | | | | |
| WISC Similarities | 32 | | | | | | |
| WISC Comprehension | 24 | 25 | | | 33 | | |
| WISC Arithmetic | 24 | | | | | 25 | 23 |
| WISC Coding | 20 | | | | | | |
| WISC Block Design | | | 21 | | | | |
| WISC Vocabulary | | 25 | 28 | | 29 | | |
| WISC Picture Arrangement | 23 | 26 | | | | | |
| Verbal IQ | 29 | 23 | 25 | | 29 | | 20 |
| Performance IQ | | 23 | | | | | |
| Full Scale IQ | 22 | 27 | 25 | | 27 | | |
| Dynamometer, right | 21 | 20 | 21 | 21 | 21 | 26 | |
| Dynamometer, left | 34 | 20 | 21 | 21 | 24 | 25 | |
| Trail Making, Part B | 29 | | 20 | 21 | | | |
| Sentence Repetition | 25 | | 23 | | | | |
| BVRT, correct | 24 | 25 | | | | | |
| BVRT, errors | 22 | | 22 | | | | |
| BVRT, distortions | 23 | 21 | | | | | |
| R-L orientation | | 23 | 30 | | | | |
| Embedded Figures, correct | | | | | | 20 | 29 |
| Writing Time, right hand | | | | 22 | | | |
| Writing Time, left hand | | | | 25 | | | |
| Tactual Performance Test time & localization | | 22 | | | | | |
| Sound Recognition Test | | | 36 | | | | |

* outcome area    1 = School Experience, 2 = Job & Employment, 3 = Learning
and Health Problems, 4 = Treatment, 5 = Social Adjustment,
6 = Personal Experience, 7 = Family & Family Relations.

and factor-weighted scores for each outcome factor were chosen. Only
variables which loaded on the representative factor with .6 or better were
included in the analysis (Table 20-5).

*Table 20-5: Canonical Correlation between Test Predictors
and Long-Term Adjustment Outcome Variables*

First Canonical Correlation: .709 Eigenvalue .503
chi-square 246.57, df 152, significance $p < .001$
Second Canonical Correlation: .566
Third Canonical Correlation: .446

Test Predictor Factors and Contribution to First and Second Canonical Correlation*

| | | | |
|---|---|---|---|
| NF 1 | Verbal Intelligence/School Achievement | .79 | -.17 |
| NF 2 | Visuo-Motor (BVRT errors & distortions) | .48 | .12 |
| NF 3 | Writing,Trail Making,Coding,Handedness | -.21 | -.06 |
| NF 4 | BVRT Rotations & Misplacements | .06 | .13 |
| NF 5 | Sex | -.11 | -.07 |
| NF 6 | Lateral Dominance, Writing Time | .21 | .95 |
| NF 7 | BVRT Rotations & Embedded Figures | .17 | .18 |
| NF 8 | Embedded Figures (Correct in Overtime) | -.05 | .07 |

Long-Term Adjustment Outcome Factors and Loadings on First and Second Canonical Correlations

| | | | |
|---|---|---|---|
| OF 1 | Adjustment Inventory Score | -.35 | -.37 |
| OF 2 | Parents Behaviour Rating & Destructiveness and Aggressiveness | -.03 | -.03 |
| OF 3 | Age at Interview and Total Number of Jobs | .44 | -.26 |
| OF 4 | School Activities and School Involvement | .35 | -.11 |
| OF 5 | Present Interaction with Sibs and Father | .17 | .10 |
| OF 6 | Personal Satisfaction and Happiness | .07 | .03 |
| OF 7 | Alcohol Use & Dating | .41 | -.18 |
| OF 8 | Parents' Rating of Affectionate Behaviour | -.28 | -.32 |
| OF 9 | Critical Judgement & Previous LD | -.16 | .26 |
| OF10 | Involvement with Police | .24 | .20 |
| OF11 | Interaction with Friends (visits, phone calls) | .17 | -.02 |
| OF12 | Intervention Recommended by Interviewer at Follow-up | -.15 | -.39 |
| OF13 | Medical Consultation | .02 | -.19 |
| OF14 | Number of Sisters | .09 | .17 |
| OF15 | Getting Along with Classmates | .16 | .26 |
| OF16 | Difficulty in Finding a Job | -.25 | .38 |
| OF17 | Preschool Attendance | -.08 | -.21 |
| OF18 | Remembers Learning Disability Well | .21 | -.18 |
| OF19 | Age when Preschool was Attended | -.09 | .15 |

* Each score represents factor weighted scores on several variables. Only variables which load on the factor represented with .6 or more are listed.

The first canonical correlation was significant with an $R$ of .709, accounting for 50.3% of the variance. This canonical correlation indicates that verbal intelligence, school achievement and visuo-motor performance were the best representatives of the test scores when related to outcome variables, and that among the outcome variables the adjustment inventory results, age at follow-up, number of jobs held, involvement in school and school activities as well as drug and alcohol use represent the first canonical outcome factors. Obviously, outcome factor 3 is age dependent: the older the subject at the time of the follow-up the more likely he was to have held more jobs. This is confirmed by other results, indicating that with increasing age our subjects showed firmer plans for the future and somewhat better occupational adjustment, but they still lagged behind their peers of 'average learners'. Another age trend was found: the older the subject, the more negatively they judged their school experience.

The discriminant function analyses reported above provide reassurance that the three LD groups were significantly different at the outset not only in terms of neurological findings, but also in their test results. The three groups still differed significantly at the time of follow-up in their late teen and early adult years in terms of reported adjustment. Moreover, they contrasted strikingly with the control group.

The analyses of predictive validity suggest a reasonably strong relationship between verbal intelligence and visuo-motor performance at age 8 to 12 and later adjustment in terms of self-report inventory scores, school involvement and activity, number of jobs held, dating, and alcohol use. These diverse areas are significantly related to test scores at time of referral. We interpret this as a demonstration of a modest degree of predictive validity of future adjustment based on these tests and accounting for approximately 50% of the variance.

*Analysis 4: Prediction of Outcome at Age 25*

Some selected results of the Phase II follow-up were submitted to a canonical analysis in order to investigate the predictive value of referral-age data for outcome at age 25. The multiple regression analyses showed that the adult WAIS-IQ was significantly related to referral-age test scores on the Benton Visual Retention Test, a composite score of Writing Time/Trailmaking/WISC-Coding/ Handedness, and the lateral dominance examination ($p < .001$), that highest salary at age 25 was significantly related to sex of subject and the Writing composite score ($p < .052$), and that level of employment at age 25 was related to the Writing composite score, Embedded Figures completed in overtime, and a composite score of Embedded Figures/Rotations on the BVRT.

The first canonical correlation between referral-age data and age-25 outcome data was .94. As in the previous analysis with age-18 variables, the WISC-VIQ, the WRAT arithmetic and reading scores, as well as the composite Writing score described above contributed to the prediction of the following outcome variables at age 25: number of grades completed in school, employment during the past 5 years, level of employment (Blishen scale coding), highest salary, and salary at the longest held job, as well as WAIS-IQ.

This analysis was based on only 38 LD subjects for whom a complete set of data was available. With this small sample the canonical correlations were not significant. A repetition of the analysis with between 89 and 163 subjects (using a pairwise deletion technique if missing data occurred) was conducted to check for major changes in the canonical analysis and for statistical significance. The first canonical correlation was .89, and the second was .71; both were significant ($p < .001$) accounting for 87% of the variance (cumulative .83 of the Eigenvaluc).

These results suggest that referral age tests retain and possibly even increase their predictive value for selected outcome variables at age 25.

Introducing sex of subject as a predictor variable into the canonical analysis provided similar results, but also a strong sex effect: females had less employment over the last 5 years, and took more academic and college courses after leaving high school.

## Analysis 5: Socio-Economic Status

A recent analysis (O'Connor & Spreen 1987) investigated the relationship between socio-economic status of parents and outcome. Previous outcome studies have differed widely in their results with the most optimistic outcome reported by studies dealing with students from private residential schools and similar priviledged educational opportunities (Bruck 1985; Childs ct al. 1982; Rawson 1968). The educational advantages provided by an affluent home and special schools as well as the assistance in job-finding by high SES parents who may have better access to community resources makes such a difference in outcome plausible.

The current study relied on students in the public school system and hence did not include children from very high SES home status; nor did it include many children from very poor SES because of the geographic location of the study. Hence, while a reasonable variability of SES is present, the range of SES was somewhat restricted.

SES was defined by four variables: father's education, mother's education, father's employment, and mother's employment (in Blishen Scale rankings, Blishen & McRoberts 1976). Outcome was defined by seven subject variables obtained during the Phase II interview: attending academic courses at college, highest grade completed at school, type of school program attended, employment during the 5 years preceding the interview at age 25, present salary, salary at the longest job held, and present employment (converted to Blishen Scale rankings).

A canonical correlation analysis investigated the multivariate relationship between the set of four predictor variables with the set of seven outcome variables to obtain an estimate of the SES effect. Mother's employment was deleted from the prediction set because of missing data and a high correlation with father's employment. The canonical correlation (adjusted) between the two sets was .526 for 65 subjects with complete data. Using the pairwise deletion technique with the total of 226 subjects, a very similar canonical correlation was obtained, strengthening the generalizability of the result. Roy's greatest characteristic root (.5699, $p < .005$) confirmed that this correlation indeed represents a single underlying dimension between the two data sets. This was confirmed by inspecting the second likelihood ratio which was not significant. Subsequent multiple regression analyses suggested that father's employment and education were the strongest contributors to the relationship.

The analysis suggests that, as expected, SES of the family home has a significant effect on outcome. Because of the somewhat restricted representation of SES in our population, the effect accounts for 28% of the outcome variance. The effect may be stronger in populations with a wider range of SES. Nevertheless, this analysis contributes to a better understanding of discrepancies between this and other outcome studies.

In *summary*, this section describes an attempt to search for differences between our three LD groups, formed on the basis of the initial neurological examination amongst the many test variables at referral age. Several of these test variables contributed to a good group discrimination which placed over 70% of the subjects into the correct group. At age 18, the outcome variables were used in a similar fashion, and again several outcome variables provided a 4-group discrimination (including controls) with over 75% correct classification; the discrimination between LD and control subjects placed over 95% of our subjects correctly.

A canonical correlation related factor scores of tests at the time of referral to factor scores of outcome at age 18. This single correlation coefficient of .709 represents an optimal expression of prediction of outcome based on referral-age tests. Another canonical analysis related the test scores at time of referral to selected outcome variables at age 25. Two canonical correlations of .89 and .71 were significant. These results suggest that, given only the referral-age test scores for LD children, approximately 50 to 87% of the outcome variance could have been predicted. This is a surprisingly proportion of the variance, considering the many other factors, e.g., socio-economic status, personality, schooling etc. which would be expected to affect outcome and which were not included in this calculation.

However, it should not be inferred that such a relationship can be predicted with certainty for the individual case. Significant predictions for groups do not imply clinical significance of prediction for the individual.

Despite a somewhat restricted range of socio-economic status in our population, SES effects were shown to account for about 28% of the outcome variance at age 25. This effect needs to be considered when other studies are reviewed who show exceptionally good outcome for LD subjects coming from affluent families or private school populations.

## 21. Specific Reading Disability, Subtypes, and Long-Term Outcome

Although the occurrence of learning disabilities (LD) in a substantial proportion of school age children (Rutter 1978) has been recognized for many decades, the investigation of specific types of LD is relatively new, based on the recognition that LD is not a homogeneous population (Benton & Pearl 1978). That reading and spelling are the major problems for most LD children has been acknowledged for some time (Orton 1937) and has led to investigations of "specific reading disability" (Bakker & Satz 1970) or developmental dyslexia and its subtypes (Satz & Morris 1981). However, reading spelling problems in the absence of impairment of other academic skills, especially arithmetic, are actually quite rare (approximately 6%, Tuokko 1982) and specific-arithmetic disabilities are even less frequent (approximately 3%).

An analysis of 102 of our subjects with complete referral test data determined whether they would be classed as specific-reading, specific-arithmetic disability or whether they were disabled in both skills at the time of referral. Cut-offs of 1 $SD$ below age and grade expectations (based on local rather than test manual norms) on either score and between the two scores were used. Six percent of the subjects were specifically impaired in reading recognition, 4% in spelling, 14% were specifically impaired in reading and spelling, 3% in arithmetic, while the remainder was impaired in both areas.

Although all subjects in this project were originally referred because of primary learning problems, a more stringent definition (achievement test scores 1 $SD$ below age and grade expectation for the referral region, i.e., urban, suburban, and rural British Columbia) confirmed that 92.1% were seriously below expectations in reading, arithmetic, or both. Subjects who met this definition of LD were tagged and some of the major analyses of the data were repeated with the 'defined LD sample' only.

At the adult level (Phase II), achievement test scores of all participants indicated that 95% were still 1 $SD$ below expected level in reading and/or arithmetic. Ten percent showed specific reading disability and 16% showed specific arithmetic disability. In a subtype analysis described later in this section, only 9 out of the first group of 63 LD children and 21 out of the second group of 96 LD children could be described as having a specific reading disability based on subtype analysis rather than specific cut-off scores.

A promising approach to the subdivision of LD comes from the inves-

91

tigation of the nature and/or cause of impairment, since it is not likely that all LD are similar in nature or result from the same cause, if indeed a cause can be identified. High-level academic skills such as reading and arithmetic can be assumed to have a finite number of component skills which may be required in combination or interaction (Applebee 1971; Shankweiler 1964), leading to the expectation of a finite number of subtypes which should be consistent and replicable across studies. Among the subtype systems proposed, a certain degree of consistency has emerged, although no general agreement on a specific system exists. One frequently used system, developed on the basis of clinical experience, is Boder's (1970) subdivision into dyseidetic, dysphonetic, and mixed types of dyslexia. Marshall and Newcombe (1973) proposed a subdivision into visual, surface and deep dyslexia based on an analysis of error types; Bakker distinguished the slow, but accurate (Type P, 'right-hemisphere strategy') from the fast, but sloppy (Type L, 'left-hemisphere strategy') reader, based on experimental studies (Bakker 1979). This is somewhat similar to Lovett's (1984) distinction between accuracy-disabled and rate-disabled readers. The two groups are expected to differ in response to different treatment strategies (Bakker 1984). Mattis, French, and Rapin (1975) derived three subtypes from an a posteriori inspection and cross-validation of their data: the primary linguistic, the articulo-graphomotor, and the visuo-perceptual type. Results similar to Mattis et al. have been reported by others based on various methods of investigation , such as cluster analysis ( Satz & Morris 1981; Lyon & Watson 1981; Watson et al. 1983); Denckla (1977) reported similar types but added a fourth (dysphonemic sequencing disorder). Decker and DeFries (1982; Decker 1982) used principal component factor scores for reading, spatial reasoning, and coding speed to classify 91% of the sample into a spatial reasoning/reading deficit, a coding speed/reading disorder, and a reading-impaired group without accompanying deficits while 9% showed impairment in all three dimensions. Subtype 3 (specific reading) showed a high degree of sibling similarity (but not similarity with parents), indicating a possible familiar mode of transmission. The use of Q-type factor analysis of LD data without preconceived groupings led Doehring and Hoshko (1977) to propose three types: associative (A), sequential (S), and oral reading disability (O), subsequently validated with discriminant analysis on a number of neuropsychological tests (accounting for 82% of their sample) (see also Doehring et al. 1981). Finally, Fisk and Rourke (1979) reported specific types of LD based on Wechsler subtest patterns within a broader test battery (see also Rourke and Strang 1983).

Not all subtypes occur with similar frequency at all ages. Doehring reported that his O-type subjects were generally younger. Satz et al. (1978) formulated a basic rule for age-related changes, documenting in his longitudinal work that younger children will present deficits basic to the reading process (i.e., in visual, sensori-motor, and cross-modal integration ability),

92

while in older children conceptual-linguistic skills are more likely to be impaired since these are the age-appropriate "primary ascendant skills". Rourke and Orr (1977), on the other hand, insisted that subtypes should persist across the school-age span. Hence, LD subtype research should take the age factor into account.

Few studies have taken a longitudinal approach to the study of LD. Satz et al. (1978) conducted a follow-up from kindergarten to grade 6. Although this study focused on early prediction, some results support the notion of age-related changes. A test of Rourke's hypothesis (Fisk & Rourke 1979) compared subtype patterns in 9-10, 11-12, and 13-14 year old children based on Q-factor analysis. Two subtypes could be found at all three age levels while the third type was not present in the youngest group and relatively few children of subtype A were found in the oldest group. It should be noted that almost half of the children in this study were sorted into residual subtypes or did not fit any of the subtypes described in the Q-factor solution. No studies have pursued the persistence of subtypes into adult age.

The present study (Haaf & Spreen 1986) allowed an investigation of three questions: (1) Can subtypes of LD in children between the ages of 8 and 12 be reliably identified and compared to previously described sub-types in the literature; (2) Is there a significant age difference in the occurrence of subtypes between younger and older children; (3) Can similar subtypes be identified in the same group of clients after longitudinal follow-up to the age of 25 years? Since neurological examination results are available for the samples used, a subsidiary question can be posed: (4) Are some subtypes more related to neurological dysfunction than others? Finally, since arithmetic achievement test data are available on our subjects, another subsidiary question (5) can be explored: does LD present as a 'specific reading disability' or as a more general deficit in one or more of the subtypes?

The analysis focused on the referral and Phase II (adult) data. Subjects were selected at both times if they had complete data for the measures used in this analysis. A referral group (Group 1, $n = 63$) and a Phase II group (Adult Group 3, $n=170$, including 46 controls) were extracted. 85.7% of the referral subjects were also present at Phase II. An additional group of referral subjects (Group 2, $n=96$) was drawn directly from the clinic files, similar to the project referral group except for a raised IQ cut-off criterion (VIQ or PIQ $> 79$) and a wider time frame for referral to provide a means for assessing possible effects of IQ on the profiles of LD samples. The group included 53.9% of the referral sample. 32.3% of this restricted IQ sample also appears in the Phase II group. Table 21-1 gives summary statistics for each of the samples. Table 21-2 lists the means for the variables used in the present study together with the regional normative means.

*Table 21-1: Summary Statistics for Samples at Time of*
*Referral and Phase II of Follow-up*

|  | LD's in Followup (Group 1) *n*=63 | LD's (Restricted IQ) (Group 2) *n*=96 | Adult LD's and Controls (Group 3) *n*=170 |
|---|---|---|---|
| Mean age |  |  |  |
| at Referral | 10.14 | 9.91 | - |
| *SD* | (1.51) | (1.89) | - |
| at Phase II |  |  | 24.28 |
| *SD* |  |  | (2.59) |
| Sex |  |  |  |
| male | 47 | 79 | 121 |
| female | 16 | 17 | 49 |
| Neurological Category (at age 8-12) |  |  |  |
| hard signs | 23 | 34 | 42 |
| soft signs | 29 | 33 | 58 |
| none | 11 | 29 | 24 |
| control | - | - | 46 |

Groups 1 and 2 were submitted to a hierarchical grouping analysis (UBC C-GROUP, Lai 1982) to determine the optimal grouping level. Ward's minimum variance technique (Ward 1963), considered to be one of the better clustering procedures available (Lorr 1983, Maxwell 1981, Rollett & Bartram 1976) was used. The two groups were analyzed separately. Variables not already in age-corrected standard scores (Sentence Repetition, Right-Left Orientation) were converted to age-appropriate standard scores with a mean of 100 and *SD* of 15, based upon regional norms for these tests (Spreen & Gaddes 1969; Gaddes & Crockett 1975).

The optimal solution was defined by observing, from the 12 cluster level downward, the jumps in the error variance index provided by the C-GROUP routine, stopping at the level before a large jump in error variance which would indicate an unwanted grouping (Mojena & Wishart 1980). A second hierarchical clustering routine (SAS CLUSTER, 1982 version) supplied an independent measure of the "cohesiveness" of the clusters (the Cubic Clustering Criterion or CCC). The solutions listed in Table 21-3 contain negative values of the CCC suggesting that the optimal solution for each sample is more heterogeneous than would be desirable (Sarle 1982).

## Table 21-2: Mean Values for Clustering Variables
### (SD in Brackets)

| Test | Group 1 LD | Group 2 Restricted IQ LD | Normative* |
|------|------------|--------------------------|------------|
| WRAT Reading | 89.1 (16.0) | 90.7 (19.3) | 115 (7.0) |
| WRAT Spelling | 87.0 (16.8) | 88.3 (19.0) | 110.5 (8.0) |
| WRAT Arithmetic | 84.0 (11.7) | 86.0 (14.5) | 103 (9.5) |
| WISC Arithmetic | 8.0 ( 2.8) | 8.4 ( 2.9) | 12.0 (3.0) |
| Similarities | 10.1 ( 3.6) | 10.5 ( 3.3) | 12.0 (3.0) |
| Vocabulary | 10.5 ( 3.3) | 10.8 ( 3.4) | 12.0 (3.0) |
| Block Design | 10.1 ( 3.2) | 10.5 ( 3.0) | 12.0 (3.0) |
| Digit Symbol | 7.8 ( 2.9) | 8.2 ( 2.9) | 12.0 (3.0) |
| Sentence Repetition | 89.4 (20.9) | 90.5 (19.9) | 100 ( 15) |
| Right-Left Orientation (Benton) | 92.4 (17.0) | 94.6 (18.0) | 100 (15) |

* Local means (British Columbia and Victoria area) for referral-age children.

| Test | Group 3 (LD Adults) | Group 3 (Control Adults) |
|------|---------------------|--------------------------|
| WRAT Reading | 49.1 (13.7)* | 67.3 (7.8)* |
| PIAT | 58.7 (14.8)* | 75.3 (7.3)* |
| WRAT Spelling | 20.5 (9.6)* | 36.3 (7.1)* |
| WRAT Arithmetic | 18.7 (5.2)* | 28.8 (5.4)* |
| WAIS Arithmetic | 7.7 (2.6) | 11.6 (2.6) |
| Similarities | 8.1 (2.9) | 11.6 (2.3) |
| Vocabulary | 7.9 (2.6) | 11.3 (2.4) |
| Block Design | 8.9 (2.9) | 12.0 (2.2) |
| Digit Symbol | 7.2 (2.4) | 11.6 (2.2) |
| Sentence Repetition | 14.7 (2.1)* | 15.6 (1.9)* |
| Word Fluency | 34.2 (10.8) | 42.9 (10.1) |
| Paired Association | 14.8 (3.5) | 18.1 (2.4) |
| Purdue Pegboard (Both Hands) | 10.8 (2.2) | 13.3 (1.7) |
| Purdue Pegboard (Assemblies) | 31.8 (7.9) | 41.7 (6.6) |
| Halstead Category Test | 31.6 (14.2) | 19.2 (12.3) |
| Right-Left Orientation (Culver) | 88.2 (42.9) | 60.9 (27.2) |

* Raw Scores. These values were not standardized to avoid unwanted ceiling effects for adult subjects.

Profiles of test means for all clusters in the two data sets were produced. Figures 21-1 and 21-2 show the means for all tests in a *z*-score format to provide better comparison between clusters in each sample. Note that a zero *z*-score reflects the mean of the LD sample, not the mean of the general population.

The selected grouping for each data set was then submitted as a starting point for a k-means iterative partitioning procedure (SAS FASTCLUS, 1982 version) to reassign any subjects inappropriatly classified (Morris, Blashfield, & Satz 1981) and search for outliers, i.e., for subjects appearing

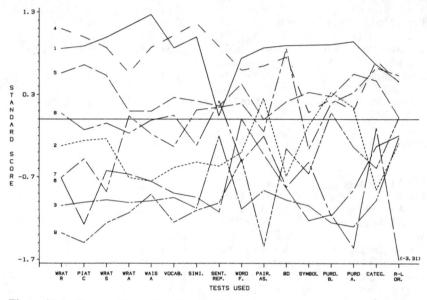

Figure 21-1 - *Z*-score Cluster Profiles for Group 1

Tests

WRAT-R - WRAT Reading
WRAT-S - WRAT Spelling
WRAT-A - WRAT Arithmetic
WISC-A - WISC Arithmetic
Sent.R. - Sentence Repetition
Simi. - WISC Similarities
Vocab. - WISC Vocabulary
BD - WISC Block Design
Cod. - WISC Coding
R-L.Or. - Right Left Orientation

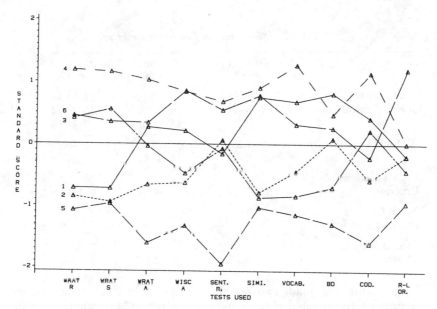

Figure 21-2 - Z-score Cluster Profiles for Group 2

Tests

WRAT-R - WRAT Reading
WRAT-S - WRAT Spelling
WRAT-A - WRAT Arithmetic
WISC-A - WISC Arithmetic
Sent.R. -    Sentence Repetition
Simi. -      WISC Similarities
Vocab. -    WISC Vocabulary
BD -          WISC Block design
Cod. -        WISC Coding
R-L.Or. -   Right Left Orientation

in clusters with an $n < 5$.

As shown in Table 21-3, several outliers appeared in groups 1 and 2, reducing slightly the percentage of subjects clustered. In each case, the number of subjects reclassified was higher than expected (group 1 = 30.2%, group 2 = 34.4%, group 3 = 34.7%). In almost all instances the reclustering appeared to split one hierarchical cluster into two iterated clusters; the largest clusters remained virtually intact. This result reflects the overall heterogeneity of some of the clusters, and again suggests caution in the interpretation of the results (Morris et al. 1981).

97

*Table 21-3: Summary of Clustering Results*

|  | Group 1 $n=63$ | | Group 2 $n=96$ | | Group 3 $n=170$ | |
|---|---|---|---|---|---|---|
| Error Variance | 8 | 14.89 | 10 | 17.69 | 11 | 31.96 |
| for Hierarchical Cluster Levels | 7 | 16.41 | 9 | 18.83 | 10 | 34.14 |
|  | 6 | 16.95 | 8 | 19.28 | 9 | 34.69 |
| (Optimal Underlined) | 5 | 21.29 | 7 | 22.40 | 8 | 40.56 |
|  | 4 | 33.02 | 6 | 28.62 | 7 | 48.29 |
| Cubic Clustering Criterion | | -2.66 | | -4.84 | | -4.26 |
| No. of Clusters (Iterated Solution) | | 6 | | 8 | | 9 |
| Percent Subjects Clustered | | 85.7 | | 91.7 | | 100 |

An attempt was made to assess the validity of the cluster solutions by comparing the iterated clusters with the results of two analyses using different algorithms, a procedure discussed by Morris et al. (1981). The SAS CLUSTER routine was repeated for groups 1 and 2 using the centroid method and average linkage on squared euclidean distances. These comparisons showed from 5% to 17% of initially grouped subjects reclustered. The small amount of reclustering shown is misleading, since the reclustering methods produced only a few large clusters in each case. For both groups, the clusters combined were those most similar in level of impairment. These results suggest that the generalizability of the grouping results is limited, although some differences between hierarchical groupings and discrete clusters should be expected (Lorr 1983).

The hierarchical solution chosen as optimal and the iterated solution (outliers removed) for both groups were submitted to a discriminant function analysis to check that the grouping level chosen is optimal as compared to other levels in the hierarchy (Doehring 1981). The analysis for group 1 showed that the hierarchical solution chosen gives only 7.9% incorrect classification, the iterated solution 13%. For group 2, the hierarchical solution produces 13.5% incorrect classification, the iterated solution 0.5%.

Analysis of variance, followed by pairwise comparisons using the *LSD* test for unequal $n$ 's (Andrews et al. 1980) if overall significance was achieved, was used to test for age effects between clusters for each solution. For the referral age group drawn from the follow-up project, the overall test for age effects failed to reach significance ($F = 1.66, p < .2$). This finding was repeated for Group 2 ($F = 0.81, p < .6$). Further analyses for age effects were therefore not considered.

98

Chi-Square analysis comparing the incidence and degree of neurological impairment for the final clusters was performed for both groups. These results were not significant for group 1 ($p < .07$) or for group 2 ($p < .2$).

To further explore the relationship between neurological impairment and subtypes, the grouping of neurological findings into five groups as described in Section 13 was used. Factor scores for each individual on the five neurological factors were compared for the nine subtypes. The MANOVA was significant ($p < .01$) and univariate tests showed that the first four factor scores provided significant group separation. As Table 21-4 shows, the mean factor scores for the two groups containing most of the control subjects (cluster 1, 4, and 5) were all low positive, as expected (negative values indicating impairment); the cluster only showing reading impairment (cluster 7) also had no distinctive neurological impairment; the two severely impaired clusters had negative factor scores on several factors; cluster 6, labelled as a visuo perceptual type, had high negative factor scores on the sensory factor 4 as well as moderately negative scores on factors 2 and 3; cluster 6, labelled as graphomotor has negative factor means on factors 1, 2, 4, and 5; the arithmetic disabled cluster 2 has negative values on factors 2, 5, and 4. These findings provide some confirmation from the neurological impairment clusters for the labels applied to the subtypes on the basis of the configuration of their test results. They suggest, for example, that the LD subtype with low visuo-perceptual test scores also had neurological impairment primarily in those parts of the physical examination which tested visual functions.

The adult group (Group 3) was analyzed using the same procedures outlined for groups 1 and 2 with the following tests: Sentence Repetition (corrected score); Word Fluency, corrected score; time score for performance of Right-Left Orientation (Culver 1969); sum of the four subtests of the shortened adult Halstead Category Test; paired associate learning (Wechsler & Stone 1945); Purdue Pegboard scores for both hands and

*Table 21-4: Mean Factor Scores for Neurological Findings for the Nine LD Subtypes*

| Cluster/Label | Factor 1 motor | Factor 2 mot./ asym. | Factor 3 mot./ speech | Factor 4 visual | Factor 5 sensory |
|---|---|---|---|---|---|
| 1 Control | .241 | .310 | .221 | .187 | .220 |
| 2 Arithmetic Disabled | .176 | -.217 | .253 | -.050 | -.138 |
| 3 Severely Impaired | .069 | -.103 | -.545 | -.098 | -.486 |
| 4 Control | .173 | .201 | .299 | .260 | .093 |
| 5 Control | .194 | .267 | .209 | .078 | .238 |
| 6 Visuo-Perceptual | -.101 | -.648 | -.669 | -1.350 | .023 |
| 7 Reading Disabled | .255 | .192 | .106 | .236 | .079 |
| 8 Graphomotor | -.600 | -.547 | .511 | -.870 | -.045 |
| 9 Severely Impaired | .524 | -.132 | -.366 | .359 | .212 |

assemblies; the reading comprehension subtest of the PIAT , raw score; raw scores for the reading, spelling and arithmetic subtests of the WRAT; scaled scores for the Similarities, Vocabulary, Digit Symbol, Block Design and Arithmetic subtests of the WAIS-R.

The data for Group 3 were not submitted to an age correction similar to Groups 1 and 2 (except for the already standardized WAIS measures) since no significant age effects for the tests have been reported in the literature for the age period from 18 to 30 years.

The hierarchical grouping analysis suggested a breakdown into 9 discrete lusters. The iterated solution also presented 9 clusters with no outliers (Figure 21-3). Since high scores indicate poor performance for the Halstead Category and timed Right-Left Orientation tests, the signs for these Z-score means were reversed in the figure. The discriminant function analysis on the hierarchical and iterated solutions showed 13.5% and 10.6% incorrect classifications, respectively.

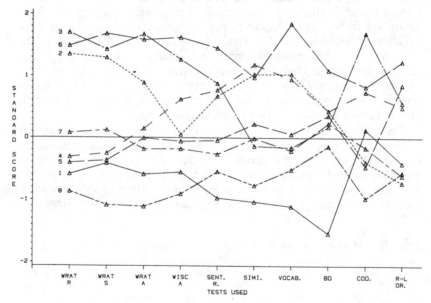

Figure 21-3 - Z-score Cluster Profiles for Group 3

The overall ANOVA for age with the adult cluster solution reached significance ($F = 3.04$, $p < .01$), and pairwise tests revealed that the two youngest and two oldest clusters were significantly different. The MANOVA on the total sample split into two groups by median age (24.7 yrs.), however, was not significant for the total sample (Wilks Lambda $F = 0.64$, $p < .9$). A stepwise multiple regression on age using the 16 clustering

100

variables resulted in two variables entering the equation, the PIAT Reading Comprehension and Word Fluency, accounting for approximately 8% of the variance. That these variables show the strongest age effects in an adult sample is perhaps not surprising, since the skills required for success continue to develop throughout the lifespan as a function of experience. Other experience-related tests, such as WAIS Vocabulary, also showed high $F$-values in the regression, but were not selected in the regression analysis.

The Chi-square analysis for degree of neurological impairment was significant (Chi-Square = 117.3, $p < .00$; Contingency Coefficient = 0.64). Subsequent inspection of the cross-tabulation revealed that the effect was primarily due to the clustering of control subjects into three clusters, and of subjects with hard neurological signs to group into one of the lowest clusters (cluster 3, Figure 21-3). That the clustering of the control subjects is the primary contributor to the significance of the Chi-square was confirmed by a reanalysis of the data with control subject groups removed (not significant, $p < .1$).

To test the validity of the solution obtained for Group 3, the SAS hierarchical routine was repeated for two random split samples ($n = 85$ each) and the results compared with the total sample solution. This replication showed that the overall solution, while still somewhat heterogeneous, was stable; each split-half solution suggested an optimal level in the same narrow range (five to seven clusters). Further, the overall pattern of the CCC was similar for both replications. The control subjects in each split-half tended to cluster in two large groups, as was the case in the analysis of the full sample. Overall, 36% of subjects did not cluster into one major cluster per subsample, though in some cases the small number of subjects present made interpretation difficult, and in only one case were the subjects in one subsample noticeably diffused. This result suggests some overall heterogeneity within clusters, but in general the cluster solution chosen seems valid.

Since outliers failed to appear in this sample, the iterated nine-cluster solution was used.

The analysis of LD clusters in this section suggests:

1. Clusters of LD in the 8-12 year old referral group of 63 children clearly show two severity-specific groups, cluster 4 ($n=8$) which was high in all performance areas, probably best described as a minimally impaired group, and cluster 5 ($n =5$) which was quite low in all areas, indicating pervasive and severe deficiency (Mean IQ=69). The small N's for these clusters suggest that these groups are composed of extreme cases not well classified otherwise, although the N's are marginally above the outlier criterion. Beyond this, one group with a profile suggesting specific arithmetic disability (group 3, $n=12$) and one group with specific reading

disability (Group 1, $n$=9) were identified. The remaining two groups (6, $n$=11, and 2, $n$=9) were impaired in all achievement areas, but differed not only in level of impairment, but also in the pattern of performance on other tests: group 6 showed more difficulties in Vocabulary, Block Design and especially in Coding, and could tentatively be labelled a visuo-perceptual (or in Boder's terminology a dyseidetic or Bakker's L) type, while group 2 showed difficulties in Similarities, Vocabulary, and Coding, and corresponds loosely to the linguistic type of Mattis. The specific reading disability group 1 shows a relative deficit in Sentence Repetition, Right-Left Orientation and to some extent in Coding, roughly corresponding to Mattis' articulo-graphomotor type (or Boder's dysphonetic type and Bakker's P).

2. For the second, larger group of 96 LD children with a more restrictive IQ criterion, again a minimally impaired group (6, $n$=6) and a severely impaired group (8, $n$=15) can be distinguished. Similar to the results for group 1, a small specific arithmetic disability group (2, $n$=6) and two specific reading impairment groups (4, $n$=10, and 5, $n$=14) are recognizable, while the remaining groups show impairment in all achievement areas. Of these, group 1 ($n$=14) is most severely impaired, but shows the lowest score on Block Design, again resembling the visuo-perceptual type; group 7 ($n$=16) shows mild impairment in most areas, but is specifically low in Right-Left Orientation, and group 3 ($n$=7) is least impaired in achievement, but shows distinct problems in Similarities and Vocabulary, resembling the linguistic type. One reading disabled group (5, $n$=14) shows problems primarily in Coding (graphomotor), while the other RD group (4, $n$=10) shows good test scores in all verbal areas, but is lowest in Block Design, Coding, and Right-Left Orientation, possibly another example of the graphomotor type.

While the cluster solutions for the two groups are not identical, the main pattern of subgroups is quite similar. Within the reading impaired groups, types emerge which resemble those proposed by Mattis and, to some extent, by Boder and Bakker. Additional subgroups are likely to occur with larger numbers of subjects as was the case in the second analysis. Moreover, the occurrence in both analyses of two subgroups differing from the others mainly in severity, both in achievement as well as other tests, is not surprising since clusters of near-normal performance and of across-the-board low performance should be expected in any grouping attempt. It should be noted that, in contrast to other studies, the clustering procedure grouped the majority of our subjects and excluded only a few outliers (see Table 21-3).

3. All 170 adult subjects were clustered (i.e., no outliers), including a group of control subjects who were normal learners when selected for the follow-up. This description of normal learners does not, of course, preclude the development of learning problems in later years, particularly

since exceptionally good learners were deliberately not included in the control sample. The 9-group clustering solution (compared to 6 and 8 for groups 1 and 2, respectively) reflects the larger number of subjects and the inclusion of the controls. LD and control group subjects differed on means for all tests used in the clustering procedure (Table 21-2b). Clusters 1 and 4 (and possibly cluster 5) in the solution (Figure 21-3) were composed mainly of control subjects (Controls/LD for cluster 1 = 26/5, cluster 4 = 9/9, cluster 5 = 9/16); only two control subjects failed to cluster into these three highest-performing groups.

Cluster 9 (n=12) seems to represent the most severely impaired group. Cluster 3 (n=21) shows good Sentence Repetition and Right Left Orientation skills, but otherwise uniform impairment, and most likely represents a second generally impaired group.

Cluster 7 (n=16) shows specific reading impairment, in combination with good performance on all other tests. Cluster 6 (n=5) shows very poor reading comprehension in the presence of good Word Fluency, poor Purdue Pegboard scores, and very poor Right-Left Orientation. This cluster might be considered a visuo-motor coordination deficit type, perhaps corresponding to the graphomotor type found among the referral-age clusters. A specific arithmetic disability is present in cluster 2 (n=25).

Cluster 8 (n=17) shows impairment in Block Design and Purdue Pegboard scores, and is possibly another example of a visuo-motor coordination deficit, but with somewhat better achievement scores and adequate reading comprehension.

The adult clusters generally tend to resemble some of the types found at middle childhood, i.e., two severely impaired groups, two specific RD groups, one arithmetic disability group and one 'mixed general impairment' group. The primarily linguistic type of impairment, however, seems to be absent at this age.

Tracing the individual subjects with data at both childhood and adult testing, Table 21-5 shows the adult clustering for the 53 group 1 subjects with a complete set of data, who participated in the 15 year follow-up.

Although the clusters at childhood do not clearly separate into corresponding clusters at adult age, some similarity is evident: cluster 3 at referral, tentatively described as an arithmetic disabled group with some impairment on verbal tasks (Figure 21-1) is best represented at adult age by cluster 2, also showing an arithmetic impairment (Figure 21-3). Further correspondence is seen between referral cluster 1, described as a reading impaired groep which seems otherwise umimpaired, and adult cluster 7, also a reading disabled group with lowest scores in Coding (Digit Symbol). Referral cluster 6, labelled a visuo-perceptual type, is best represented by adult cluster 8, with low scores also in the nonverbal measures (including visuo-motor tests such as the Purdue tasks which were not available at referral age). This referral cluster (6) also seems to be represented in part by

Table 21-5: Number of Subjects in Corresponding Subtypes at
Referral Age (Group 1) and Adult Age (Group 3)

| Referral Clusters | 1 | 2 | 3 | 4 | 5 | 6 | O* |
|---|---|---|---|---|---|---|---|
| Adult Clusters | | | | | | | |
| 1 | 1 | | | 1 | | | |
| 2 | 1 | 2 | 6 | 1 | | 1 | |
| 3 | | 3 | 2 | | 2 | | 1 |
| 4 | | | | | | 3 | 1 |
| 5 | 1 | | | 1 | | 2 | 3 |
| 6 | | | | | 1 | | |
| 7 | 4 | 1 | | 1 | | 1 | 1 |
| 8 | | | 3 | | | 4 | |
| 9 | | 2 | | | 1 | | 2 |

* Outliers

adult cluster 4, a relatively nonimpaired cluster (50% controls) with a similar pattern on nonverbal tests (Figure 21-3). It should also be noted that the majority of outliers in the group 1 analysis appear in adult clusters 5 (a relatively nonimpaired group) and 9 (the lowest achievement-test group). In total, 19 out of 53 subjects appear in similar disability subgroups at both childhood and adult age.

4. A test of the age differentiation hypothesis for the referral age samples was not significant, indicating that the hypothesis of certain subtype clusters appearing more often in younger or older children cannot be confirmed with the current sample in the age range from 8 to 12 years. The data for the referral age groups were submitted to an age correction before analysis, and it is suggested that such a procedure be followed in future studies of subtype age differences to avoid the confounding aspects of raw scores which may cluster along a severity continuum directly related to age.

5. The Chi-Square analysis investigating the association between LD subtypes and neurological impairment (hard or soft neurological signs) was not significant for the referral age groups, suggesting that none of the qualitative and severity-related subtypes discussed above are specifically associated with neurological impairment. A similar analysis for the adult subjects was significant; however, this was the result of the emergence of discrete control subject clusters. Since all control subjects were automatically assigned an impairment category of 4 (nonimpaired) for initial neurological status, this result simply reiterates the LD-control severity distinction. As in the referral age clusters, neurological impairment in childhood does not appear to be significantly related to LD clustering in adulthood. This question was explored further for the adult group by performing a second Chi-Square analysis between cluster membership and neurological status as measured by a follow-up neurological examination

at Phase II. All subjects, including controls, were assigned to either a 'hard-sign', 'soft-sign' or a 'no-sign' neurological group (Hern 1984). At this time, several control subjects were found to belong in the 'soft-sign' group. The Chi-Square analysis with all clusters was significant ($p < .000$). Again, the three control subject clusters contained the majority of 'soft-sign' and 'no-sign' subjects (and no subjects with hard signs). With the control subject groups removed, this analysis remained significant ($p < .02$). Further inspection revealed that cluster 3, described as a generally impaired group, included the largest number of hard-sign subjects, and no subjects in the 'no-sign' group. The same pattern was seen in cluster 6, described as a possible visuo-motor deficit type with very poor scores on some tests. A pattern similar to that of the control groups was seen in cluster 7, where no subjects with hard signs were present (this group was described as a reading-disabled subtype with good overall test scores). In general, it seems that, when the adult subject's neurological status is reassessed, a relationship is found between degree of neurological impairment and the severity dimension of the clustering results.

6. In an additional analysis, one often-reported LD subtype, referred to as the 'ACID' subtype, was specifically searched for in the present data. This subtype has been defined as showing low scores on the WISC Arithmetic, Coding, Information, and Digit Span subtests, with all other scores not impaired (Rourke & Strang 1983, Rourke 1985). Subjects with scaled scores for all subtests of the WISC or WAIS were drawn from referral ($n = 90$) and Phase II ($n = 188$, 51 controls) of the follow-up project.

These data were submitted to an hierarchical grouping procedure, and the optimal solution iteratively searched as described previously. The adult group was first analyzed with the control subjects removed, then with the controls added to investigate any possible changes in clustering. Table 21-6 presents the summary statistics for these groups and an outline of the results obtained.

All relevant cluster profiles are shown in Table 21-7 with the scaled subtest scores.

The cluster profiles for the referral age sample showed two subgroups which correspond to the ACID type. The best fitting ACID group (where all non-ACID subtests are close to the mean of 10) accounted for 19% of the sample ($n = 17$). A second group also showed the ACID pattern ($n = 32$, 36% of sample), but all subtest scores were low, with the four relevant tests being the lowest overall. This suggests that this group is more uniformly disabled than is expected of a distinct syndrome, and so perhaps should not be considered as a clear example of the ACID type.

The profiles of the full adult group (control subjects excluded) show one cluster corresponding to the ACID subtype ($n = 24$, 12.4% of sample), with all other scores except Vocabulary close to or above the mean. The profiles of the adult group with the control subjects included show the controls

*Table 21-6: Summary Statistics for Samples used in ACID Subtype Analysis*

|  | Referral Age (*n*=90) | Adult Age (*n*=137) | Adult Age (Including Controls) (*n*=188) |
|---|---|---|---|
| Mean age (SD) | | | |
| At Referral | 9.91 (1.47) | - | - |
| At Phase II | - | 24.3 (2.70) | 24.3 (2.60) |
| Mean IQ | 97.4 | 86.9 | 93.2 |
| Sex | | | |
| Male | 64 | 101 | 133 |
| Female | 26 | 36 | 55 |
| Neurological Category (At age 8-12) | | | |
| hard signs | 29 | 53 | 53 |
| soft signs | 40 | 59 | 59 |
| none | 21 | 25 | 25 |
| control | - | - | 51 |
| No. of Clusters (Hierarchical) | 5 | 7 | 9 |
| Cubic Clustering Criterion | -3.24 | -5.10 | -4.66 |
| No. of Clusters (Iterated) | 5 | 6 | 9 |
| Percent Subjects Clustered | 100 | 91.2 | 96.3 |

clustering almost entirely (82.4%) in three additional clusters, with only 13.7% of control subjects entering other clusters. This indicates that their inclusion adds only minimal distortion to the solution for LD subjects, as was the case in the previous analyses. Two groups displaying an ACID syndrome appear, the best fitting ACID group (*n*=17) comprised largely (75.9%) of control subjects. This cluster accounts for 9% of the total sample. The second adult ACID group (*n*=25) consists of LD subjects, and two controls (13.3% of sample). Again, the overall pattern of performance is low, suggesting that this group is more representative of a 'general LD' subtype.

Tracing referral-age subjects in the distinct ACID cluster to adult clusters shows that 4 of 17 (23.5%) subjects enter the adult ACID cluster; 5 of 17 (29.4%) enter an adult cluster showing overall low performance (below

| | Referral | | Adult LD | Adult Full Sample | |
|---|---|---|---|---|---|
| | CL3 (17) | CL4 (32) | CL3 (24) | CL5 (17) | CL8 (25) |
| Information | 8.82 | 6.47 | 8.25 | 11.82 | 7.56 |
| Picture Completion | 14.06 | 8.03 | 11.54 | 12.71 | 10.72 |
| Similarities | 11.70 | 7.19 | 9.21 | 13.53 | 7.96 |
| Picture Arrangement | 11.12 | 7.41 | 11.33 | 12.53 | 11.04 |
| Arithmetic | 7.82 | 6.34 | 8.50 | 11.88 | 7.32 |
| Block Design | 10.18 | 7.94 | 10.67 | 12.94 | 8.92 |
| Vocabulary | 11.35 | 7.91 | 8.92 | 12.88 | 7.88 |
| Object Assembly | 12.53 | 7.78 | 9.96 | 12.77 | 8.08 |
| Comprehension | 9.35 | 7.38 | 10.08 | 13.65 | 9.52 |
| Coding/Digit Symbol | 9.00 | 6.44 | 7.29 | 10.12 | 7.84 |
| Digit Span | 7.00 | 6.06 | 7.71 | 11.71 | 7.60 |

8.60 on all subtests). The remaining ACID subjects are dispersed throughout the solution (four were not followed up). Tracing these subjects into the second adult solution (including controls), shows 5 of 17 (29.4%) entering the adult low-performance ACID cluster (8), and no referral-age ACID subjects entering the ACID cluster consisting mainly of control subjects; four subjects were again not followed up, and the remaining referral subjects were dispersed throughout the solution.

These results indicate that, while good examples of the ACID subtype can be found at both ages, overall severity must be considered in the selection of interpretable clusters. That such a subtype appears at adult age in clusters comprised largely of average learners suggests that the ACID LD subtype may not persist into adulthood and is specific to middle childhood; alternatively, this subtype may be viewed as common among adults without specific LD history.

7. A supplementary analysis of the present data for adult subjects was suggested by the findings of Aylward (1984), who investigated visual and auditory lateralization across reading-disability subtypes. She reported an exaggerated right-ear advantage for dichotic listening in such subtypes when compared to normal readers, suggesting that this may reflect exaggerated perceptual asymmetry in dyslexic subjects that is the result of attentional deficits. To investigate this hypothesis on adult subjects and with empirically derived subtypes, a similar analysis was performed on the dichotic listening test data collected at Phase II. The nine-cluster solution for the 170 adult subjects was used; all subjects had valid dichotic listening data except for one subject who was excluded due to a severe hearing

impairment in the right ear. Mean right and left ear scores for each cluster are presented in Table 21-8.

*Table 21-8: Mean Right and Left Ear Dichotic Listening*
*Scores for Adult Subjects (n=169)*

| Mean(SD) | Right Ear | Left Ear |
|---|---|---|
| 1(31) | 29.45 | 20.48 |
| | (5.81) | (6.75) |
| 2(25) | 26.40 | 15.84 |
| | (9.26) | (9.27) |
| 3(20) | 28.40 | 10.45 |
| | (9.28) | (7.13) |
| 4(18) | 29.28 | 22.44 |
| | (6.52) | (7.57) |
| 5(25) | 30.64 | 20.76 |
| | (5.78) | (6.87) |
| 6(05) | 20.20 | 16.60 |
| | (12.68) | (8.62) |
| 7(16) | 28.13 | 18.69 |
| | (8.02) | (5.64) |
| 8(17) | 31.06 | 14.47 |
| | (9.22) | (9.79) |
| 9(12) | 24.42 | 12.92 |
| | (6.39) | (5.76) |

For each subject a laterality index (LI) was calculated, based upon the formula proposed by Marshall et al. (1975) and used by Aylward:

$$\text{Total Accuracy } 50\%, \text{LI} = \text{Rc - Lc} / \text{Rc + Lc}$$
$$\text{Total Accuracy } 50\%, \text{LI} = \text{Rc - Lc} / \text{Re + Le}$$

Where Rc = total correct right ear, Re = total errors right ear, Lc = total correct left ear and Le = total errors left ear. The formula is designed to compensate for the negative bias that occurs when the difference score is divided by the total number of correctly repeated words.

Analysis of variance for unequal $n$'s was performed across clusters, and overall significance was achieved ($F = 2.24, p < .05$). Pairwise comparisons using the LSD test revealed that clusters 3 and 8, with the largest positive mean scores indicating right-ear preference (0.455 and 0.382 respectively, compared to 0.208 for the highest-scoring control cluster 5), were the only groups significantly different from the other clusters. These clusters seem to represent a generally impaired type (cluster 3) and a visuo-spatial or visuo-motor type (cluster 8); the strongest right-ear effect occurs in cluster 3. This suggests that the exaggerated right-ear preference is present, but does not necessarily occur in the specific reading-disabled groups.

In *summary*, the replication of previously described types of LD was partially successful. Previous studies have shown some consensus in describing a visuo-perceptual, a linguistic and an articulo-graphomotor type. Although the tests selected for this analysis differed substantially from those of other authors, all three types were identified in two separate cluster analyses of 8- to 12-year old LD children. In addition, the occurrence of a minimally impaired and a severely impaired group was noted.

While other authors have specified reading as the primary impairment of their LD subjects (but without providing data on other types of academic achievement) the inclusion of two measures of arithmetic achievement confirmed that only relatively few LD subjects can be characterized as having "specific" reading impairment, and even fewer as having "specific" arithmetic impairment, while the majority of subjects showed impairment in both achievement areas.

The exploration of clusters in the same subject population with a restricted-IQ sample and in an adult sample including average learners ('controls') after a 15-year interval addressed a question which so far has not been investigated. The cluster analysis suggests that the average learners can be readily distinguished from the LD group on all measures, including academic achievement. Three clusters at adult age represented mainly control subjects, and one cluster a severely impaired group. Among the remaining clusters, only the visuo-perceptual and the graphomotor types could be identified, while the linguistic-impairment subtype was no longer recognizable. LD subjects displaying a visuo-spatial deficit at childhood maintain their impairment over this age span, and reading and arithmetic problems persist into adult age. Severely impaired and nonimpaired performance also seem to continue in some subjects, but the subjects of a subgroup with linguistic impairment appeared in overall low-performance adult clusters, perhaps suggesting a poor long-term outcome. This result seems to support in general the prediction that such deficits worsen in the early adult years (e.g. Gottesman et al. 1975), and contradict the primary ascendant skill hypothesis of Satz. It must be stressed, however, that Satz's hypothesis does not extend into the late teen and early adult period. It may well be that children with primary linguistic impairment at age 8-12 never 'catch up' and so develop into a generally impaired subtype in the early adult years, while other, more pervasive deficits such as visuo-motor or visuo-spatial problems severe enough to persist into age 8-12, could maintain a distinct pattern.

A search for Rourke's ACID subtype suggested that this form of LD occurs with a limited frequency both at childhood and adult age. However, in our sample little persistence of the ACID subtype into adulthood could be found; in fact, several control subjects displayed this disability pattern.

No confirmation was found for Aylward's hypothesis that specific reading-disabled subjects show an exaggerated right-ear preference in dichotic listening.

109

## 22. Outcome for Children Described as Hyperactive

Hyperkinesis, hyperactivity, or attention deficit disorder has been the subject of a number of follow-up studies (Ackerman, Dykman, & Peter 1977a, b; Loney et al. 1984). The studies of Weiss collaborators (Weiss et al. 1971; Werry et al. 1972; Minde et al. 1971, 1972; Hechtman et al. 1976), by Cordoni et al. (1981), and by Mendelson et al.1971) and Menkes et al. (1967) in particular, have pointed out that hyperactive children do not simply 'grow out' of their difficulties, but continue to present a changing set of problems as adolescents and adults, although delinquency and psychosis are rare. A reevaluation of 75 of the original group of 104 adolescents and 45 controls at the age of 17 to 25 by Weiss showed longer periods of drug use and an older age at discontinuation of drugs such as stimulants, hashish, and marijuana, although recent use was not significantly different from controls; alcohol was more heavily used; aggression as a problem in the individual's history occurred more often, more severely, and at a slightly younger age; court referrals were more frequent, but not significantly so; thefts of items valued at more than $ 500 occurred in 6 subjects and none of the controls; no differences were found on Kohlberg's test of moral judgement. Loney et al. (1984) were specifically investigating the potential predictors of outcome with multivariate techniques. They point out that childhood symptom dimensions such as aggressiveness, and socio-ecological environmental measures such as parenting style have been predictors of adolescent symptoms (a point also stressed, perhaps excessively, by Lewis & Balla 1976). Loney found that paternal control, aggression-factor scores, and the presence of neurological signs all contributed to a multiple regression analysis of 'offenses against persons', while involvement with illegal drugs at adolescent follow-up was predicted to some degree by the aggression-factor score, age at referral, urban residence, and response to drug treatment in hyperactive children. Finally, Borland and Heckman (1976) found lower socio-economic achievement status in former ADS adults as compared to their siblings, although they seemed to achieve adequately socially and occupationally. The study also suggests that subjects with persisting symptoms of hyperactivity as adults did not show poorer outcome than adults without persisting symptoms.

For the analysis in our current study all information pertaining to the hyperactivity-attention deficit complex of behaviour was reviewed. The interviewer rated each individual on his/her ability to concentrate at the time of Phase I. A 3-point rating was labelled as average while a rating of 1 indicated that the individual 'persisted beyond the need to continue, cannot shift to other activites' and a 6-point rating referred to being 'unable to attend to the task, distracted by own ideas'. The four groups differed significantly on this rating in a linear fashion (3.16, 3.49, 2.88, and

2.78 respectively; $p < .01$). During the Phase II interview the same ratings were made and similar findings obtained (2.88, 2.94, 2.92 and 2.62 respectively; $p < .05$). Males received significantly poorer ratings than females.

The parents rated their children on a similar scale for "attentiveness," 'impulsivity' of the child, destructiveness, activity level ('on the go'), the tendency to get into arguements and fights, and the tendency towards negativism or contrariness. All of these ratings show a significant group difference between LD and controls. Group 3 showed the most negative rating on several of the scales (Table 22-1). Sex differences on these variables were not significant.

*Table 22-1:Percent Ratings of Participants at Phase I Interview for Attention Span, Impulsiveness, Destructiveness, and Energy Level by Group\**

| Group | 1 | 2 | 3 | Control | $p<$ |
|---|---|---|---|---|---|
| *Characteristic Rated* | | | | | |
| Attention Span | 3.03 | 3.22 | 3.08 | 2.63 | .016 |
| Impulsiveness | 3.69 | 3.49 | 3.39 | 2.73 | .002 |
| Destructiveness | 2.08 | 1.84 | 2.18 | 1.39 | .090 |
| Energy Level | 3.87 | 4.13 | 4.69 | 4.58 | .060 |
| Fighting & Arguements | 2.84 | 2.81 | 3.09 | 2.07 | .002 |
| Negativism & Contrariness | 3.02 | 2.86 | 3.18 | 2.43 | .050 |

\* low ratings represent the positive and high ratings the negative end of each scale.

The participants were asked during Phase II of the study whether they had ever been characterized as hyperactive. Twenty-seven percent of our subjects said 'yes', but the majority of these subjects were in group 3, and the smallest number in the control group (24.1, 33.9, 50.0, and 11.8 respectively; $p < .002$). A similar finding was obtained, when subjects during the Phase II interview were asked whether they often felt restless (42.3, 48.1, 53.8, and 25.0 respectively; $p < .07$).

A related question addressed behaviour problems of our subjects. Asked during Phase I whether they or their parents considered them to have a behaviour problem before the time of the initial referral, almost 40% said yes (54.2, 38.7, 46.2, and 24.0 respectively; $p < .02$) and 50% described themselves as having a behaviour problem (including anxiety, acting out behaviour, destructiveness, temper tantrums, etc.) after the initial referral (59.4, 55.9, 56.5, and 26.1% respectively; $p < .002$).

These related variables were factor analyzed (Table 22-2) resulting in three major factors: impulsivity/negativity, temper/fighting, and hyperactivity/behaviour problems. An additional 'concentration' factor was also present. These factors seem to correspond to other factors described for behaviour problems of children, e.g. inconsequence/unforthcomingness,

111

*Table 22-2: Factor Analysis of ADS Problems Reported by*
*Parents and Subjects*

| | Factor 1 impulsivity/ negativity | Factor 2 temper/ fighting | Factor 3 hyperactive/ beh.problem | Factor 4 concen- tration |
|---|---|---|---|---|
| Concentration | .18901 | -.01857 | .03490 | .88816 |
| Fighting | .43292 | .73850 | .04800 | -.08583 |
| Temper Outbursts | .29339 | .82908 | .13389 | .02532 |
| Energy Level | .28980 | -.57688 | .20002 | -.45371 |
| Impulsivity | .71419 | .25308 | .12881 | .06101 |
| Attentiveness | .72118 | .07520 | .26321 | .13230 |
| Destructiveness | .77641 | .09693 | -.04196 | .04944 |
| Contrariness, Negativism | .62929 | .42210 | .10453 | -.08068 |
| Behaviour Problems in Childhood | .32401 | .09892 | .58262 | -.01071 |
| Later Behaviour Problems | .30254 | .41025 | .42832 | -.03085 |
| Hyperactivity | .02850 | .02887 | .77371 | -.21081 |
| Restlessness | -.03070 | -.01805 | .71600 | .20883 |

hostility/peer maladaptiveness and a general overreaction factor described by McDermott (1981); her general underreaction factor, however, was not present in this analysis. This may be due to the use of structured interview and parent rating items rather than the Revised Bristol Adjustment Guides (for teachers) used by McDermott. The variables from the preceding analysis were included in a four-group discriminant function analysis in order to determine how well the groups could be separated on the basis of these personality characteristics alone. Table 22-3 indicates that restlessness and behaviour problems separated the four groups to a significant degree.

However, even after inclusion of all six significant variables, the group separation between groups 2 and 3 remained nonsignificant and the overall group classification rate was only 46.7% correct, suggesting that groups were significantly different, but not adequately separated with these variables.

All subjects were reclassified into 'hyperactive' and 'nonhyperactive' on the basis of a score derived from the addition of the hyperactivity and concentration scores. This score was significantly different across the four groups (59.7, 67.1, 85.7, and 31.4% respectively; chi-square = 28.53, $p <$ .000), confirming the results described above. A second analysis based on rated activity level during adolescence as provided by the parents during the Phase I interview (Table 22-4) provided further support.

An attempt was made to relate presence or absence of hard and soft neurological findings at Phase II follow-up to the degree of hyperactivity (Table 22-5). The neurological findings were only marginally related to

*Table 22-3: Discriminant Function Between the Four Groups on Variables Relating to the Hyperactivity/Attention Deficit Syndrome*

|  |  | Degrees of Freedom | | Significance |
|---|---|---|---|---|
| Wilks' Lambda | 0.705719 | 2 | 3 | 122.0 |
| Equivalent $F$ | 7.678490 |  | 6 | 242.0 | 0.0000 |

Variables in the Analysis After Step 2

| Variable | Tolerance | $F$ to Remove | Wilks' Lambda |
|---|---|---|---|
| "On-the-go" | 0.9521535 | 6.4653 | 0.8188428 |
| Behaviour problems subsequent to first referral | 0.9521535 | 10.859 | 0.8957196 |

| Group | 1 | 2 | 3 |
|---|---|---|---|
| **Group** |  |  |  |
| 2 | 3.1676 |  |  |
|  | 0.0456 |  |  |
| 3 | 4.0117 | 1.8457 |  |
|  | 0.0206 | 0.1623 |  |
| Control | 20.784 | 8.0193 | 5.0879 |
|  | 0.0000 | 0.0005 | 0.0076 |

*Results of Group Classification by Discriminant Function Analysis With Hyperactivity Variables Only*

Classification Results

| Actual Group | No. of Cases | Predicted Group Membership | | | |
|---|---|---|---|---|---|
|  |  | 1 | 2 | 3 | Control |
| 1 | 45 | 23 | 12 | 1 | 9 |
|  |  | 51.1% | 26.7% | 2.2% | 20.0% |
| 2 | 48 | 16 | 11 | 2 | 19 |
|  |  | 33.3% | 22.9% | 4.2% | 39.6% |
| 3 | 14 | 2 | 3 | 3 | 6 |
|  |  | 14.3% | 21.4% | 21.4% | 42.9% |
| Control | 45 | 3 | 8 | 0 | 34 |
|  |  | 6.7% | 17.8% | 0.0% | 75.6% |

Percent of "Grouped" Cases Correctly Classified: 46.71%

hyperactivity in childhood. The relationship was more clearly established in males compared to females.

In an attempt to analyze the effect of this 'activity' score on type of employment, the jobs reported by participants were reclassified as either providing 'active' (trades, unskilled labor, sales) or less active (clerical, professional, sedentary) types of work. The four groups differed significantly on active vs. nonactive jobs, with the highest number of active

*Table 22-4: Percent of Subjects Classified by Activity Level
in 3 LD Groups and Controls as Related to Neurological
Impairment in Childhood*

| Group | Learning | Disabled | | Control |
|---|---|---|---|---|
| | Hard | Soft | No | No |
| | Neurological Signs | | | |
| Degree of Activity | | | | |
| 1(low) | 23 | 23 | 11 | 42 |
| 2 | 28 | 32 | 12 | 28 |
| 3 | 35 | 37 | 8 | 19 |
| 4 | 32 | 36 | 25 | 8 |

chi square $= 27.59, p < .001$

*Table 22-5: Neurological Findings at Age 25 at Four Levels of
Activity during Childhood and Adolescence*

| Neurological Activity Level | None | Soft | Hard |
|---|---|---|---|
| 1 (low) | 14 | 19 | 29 |
| 2 | 21 | 21 | 19 |
| 3 | 41 | 22 | 12 |
| 4 | 24 | 37 | 39 |

chi square $= 9.91, p < .12$

males only

| | | | |
|---|---|---|---|
| 1 (low) | 14 | 19 | 32 |
| 2 | 24 | 23 | 12 |
| 3 | 43 | 20 | 8 |
| 4 | 19 | 39 | 48 |

chi square $= 12.64 , p < .049$

jobs in Group 3 (Table 22-6). However, this difference, based on the job descriptions given at age 18, was no longer significant when applied to job descriptions at age 25.

The overall job and employment situation of our subjects in relation to hyperactivity was assessed by a discriminant function analysis, using the major variables described in Section 8. A significant group separation was already obtained with the first variable entered (Table 22-7) indicating that there was a significant difference in employment between hyperactive and

114

*Table 22-6: Percentage of Participants Holding 'Active' Types*
*Jobs at Age 19 and Age 25 Interview*

| Group | Learning Disabled | | | Control | | |
|---|---|---|---|---|---|---|
| | Hard | Soft | No | No | | |
| | Neurological Signs | | | | chi-square | p |
| Phase I | 40.0 | 37.9 | 50.0 | 17.8 | 9.144 | .027 |
| Phase II | 24.5 | 34.5 | 33.3 | 39.1 | 2.452 | ns |

*Table 22-7: Discriminant Function of Hyperactive Versus*
*Nonhyperactive Subjects on Job and Employment Variables*

| | | Degrees of Freedom | | Significance | |
|---|---|---|---|---|---|
| Wilks' Lambda | 0.834104 | 6 | 1 | 102.0 | |
| Equivalent $F$ | 3.215403 | | 6 | 97.0 | 0.0064 |

Variables in the Analysis After Step 8

| Variable | Tolerance | $F$ to Remove | Wilks' Lambda |
|---|---|---|---|
| Employment Source of | 0.9572804 | 1.6119 | 0.8479652 |
| Income Salary at Last | 0.6806185 | 2.4996 | 0.8555987 |
| of Current Job Currently | 0.6957606 | 1.9041 | 0.8504775 |
| Employed Type of | 0.9495334 | 4.9975 | 0.8770779 |
| Current Job Total Number of Jobs held in | 0.9533881 | 1.5442 | 0.8473831 |
| Last 5 Years | 0.7805157 | 4.5699 | 0.8734008 |

| Group | 1 |
|---|---|
| Group 2 | 3.2154 |
| | 0.0064 |

*Classification of Hyperactive and Non-Hyperactive Subjects*
*based on Job and Employment Variables*

| Actual Group | No. of Cases | Predicted Group 1 | Membership 2 |
|---|---|---|---|
| 1 | 77 | 57 | 10 |
| | | 87% | 13% |
| 2 | 54 | 31 | 23 |
| | | 57.4% | 42.6% |
| Ungrouped Cases | 21 | 16 | 5 |
| | | 76.2% | 23.8% |

Percent of 'Grouped' Cases Correctly Classified: 68.70%

nonhyperactive subjects. The full range of employment variables provided a highly significant group separation, but the overall correct classification rate was only 68.7%. This suggests again that presence or absence of hyperactivity has a significant effect on success in jobs and employment, but that group membership prediction remains at a relatively low level.

Since Loney et al. (1983) reported a relationship between hyperactivity (interpreted as MBD by the authors and based on whether or not the child had been referred to and included in a stimulant drug treatment program at the University of Iowa) and both delinquency and drug abuse during the teenage years, a reanalysis of the relevant data in our study was made, although our hyperactivity index, of course, does not approximate the selection criteria of the Iowa study.

To redefine the term 'hyperactive' with the information available for our subjects, the activity index described above was used; in addition, a very low, low, medium, high and very high active group assignment was created by using retrospective parent and student ratings for 'ability to concentrate, tendency towards fighting with others, temper outbursts, impulsivity, destructiveness, 'contrariness', and restlessness. In addition, drug use data were summed for prescribed and street drugs, and frequency of use.

The analyses indicated that the activity index was significantly related to membership in LD and control groups (higher activity level in all three LD groups, especially in group 2, SBD, $p < .0001$). For the total street drug use only one significant group difference emerged (39, 37, and 17% of groups 1, 2 and 3 did not use these drugs at all, while only 6.8% of controls did not use them). Similarly, more subjects in the three LD groups said they had used no prescribed drugs compared to controls, although, at the same time, a small percentage of subjects, especially in group 2, reported frequent use of such drugs (significant only in males, $p < .02$).

Using several varying definitions of the hyperactivity index, a significantly higher use of street drugs or prescribed drugs by high active-rated subjects emerged; significant differences seemed to point towards more use of street drugs by high and middle active groups, while minimal and low active groups showed lower use figures (both in males and females, Table 22-8).

No relationship between activity level and alcohol use could be established, although the high active subjects did admit more often that, at least sometimes, alcohol use lead to problems in their life (Table 22-9). This difference was no longer present at age 25.

Hence, our results provide some qualified support for Loney's findings with regard to alcohol and drug use. It should be noted, however, that only alcohol problems, not alcohol use frequencies, differed significantly with level of activity. Similarly, use of over-the-counter and prescription drugs did not differ significantly.

The relationship between activity level and delinquency was explored in

116

### Table 22-8: Total Street Drug Use at Three
### Levels of Activity at Age 19

| Street Drug Use | Activity Level | | |
|---|---|---|---|
| | low | medium | high |
| none | 15 | 18 | 0 |
| rare | 55 | 41 | 9 |
| medium | 24 | 18 | 72 |
| frequent | 6 | 24 | 18 |

chi square $= 22.30, p < .001$

### Table 22-9: Alcohol-Related Problems at Four Levels of ADS

| activity level | Age 19 | | | | Age 25 | | | |
|---|---|---|---|---|---|---|---|---|
| | low | moderate | medium | high | low | moderate | medium | high |
| never | 94 | 87 | 63 | 73 | 92 | 94 | 79 | 77 |
| sometimes | 4 | 9 | 32 | 19 | 4 | 6 | 21 | 17 |
| frequently | 1 | 2 | 0 | 5 | 4 | 0 | 0 | 5 |
| always | 0 | 2 | 5 | 3 | 4 | 0 | 0 | 1 |

chi square $= 20.02, p < .018$          chi square $= 9.11, p < .43$

several analyses and also brought only limited support for Loney's findings. Significant differences between groups with different levels of activity were found for the percent of subjects with police contacts ('did you come to the attention of the police') at the Phase I, but not the Phase II interview (Table 22-10).

Also, the number of offenses reported at the Phase I, but not the Phase II interview, and the total number of offenses reported in both interviews, differed significantly (Table 22-11). Penalties did not differ significantly between activity level groups.

### Table 22-10: Percent of Subjects who Came to the Attention
### of the Police at Phase I Interview by Activity Level

| Actitivity Level | low | medium | high | chi-square | $p <$ |
|---|---|---|---|---|---|
| Age 19 | 52 | 62 | 91 | 6.00 | .05 |
| Age 25 | 55 | 50 | 82 | 3.49 | .17 |

chi square $= 6.00, p < .05$

Table 22-11: Offenses at Age 19, Age 25 and Total Offenses
by Activity Level

| | Age 19 Offenses | | | Age 25 Offenses | | | Total Offenses | | |
|---|---|---|---|---|---|---|---|---|---|
| Activity level | low | medium | high | low | medium | high | low | medium | high |
| No. of Offenses | | | | | | | | | |
| 0 | 51 | 41 | 9 | 45 | 15 | 18 | 26 | 29 | 0 |
| 1 | 31 | 23 | 27 | 22 | 15 | 18 | 33 | 9 | 9 |
| 2 | 3 | 18 | 18 | 9 | 3 | 9 | 3 | 15 | 0 |
| 3 | 4 | 3 | 18 | 12 | 9 | 0 | 16 | 6 | 18 |
| 4 | 10 | 15 | 27 | 12 | 23 | 54 | 4 | 15 | 9 |
| 5 or more | 0 | 0 | 0 | 0 | 0 | 0 | 16 | 26 | 63 |
| chi square = | 16.81 | | | 14.39 | | | 36.94 | | |
| $p <$ | .03 | | | .07 | | | .00 | | |

In *summary*, a variety of self-report, parent- and interviewer-ratings related to the attention deficit syndrome showed differences between LD and control subjects. High ratings were not clearly related to neurological impairment, but were more often found in the LD group without neurological findings. Four different ADS factors were extracted, but group membership dicrimination based on these factors was poor, though significant. An activity level classification provided better results which were related to degree of neurological impairment in males.

It should be remembered that this study was targeted on the outcome of LD, not of children primarily referred because of ADS. With this target group, children ranked along a factor-analytically validated ADS dimension as high tended to show more neurological findings, had more active types of jobs, used more street drugs, had more problems with alcohol, and reported a higher degree of delinquency than low ADS participants at the age 19 follow-up, although discrimination between high and low ADS groups on these variables was not as powerful as might have been expected. At the second follow-up at age 25, most of these relationships were no longer significant, although trends persisted.

Rather than interpret these findings as evidence of problems continuing into adult life, as some authors have suggested, our results would support a gradually diminishing role of the ADS in an LD population as they grow into adulthood. Other factors, e.g., neurological impairment, school achievement, personality, and intelligence would seem to remain much more influential in comparison.

## 23. Test Reliability over Fifteen Years.

The retesting of our participants at Phase II provided an opportunity to investigate the long-term reliability of a limited number of tests (Sarazin & Spreen, 1986). Alternatively, the results of re-testing may also be viewed as indicators of trait stability in our participants. A total of 133 subjects were available for test-retest comparison although not all subjects had taken all tests at time 1. The correlation coefficients for all tests given on both occasions are summarized in Table 23-1.

*Table 23-1: Correlation Coefficients for Corresponding Tests Given at a Mean Age of 10 and 25 Years in LD Subjects*

| Test | All Ss | n | BD | n | MBD | n | LD | n |
|---|---|---|---|---|---|---|---|---|
| Category Test Int/Adult | .473 | 64 | .473 | 26 | .547 | 30 | .589 | 8 |
| Category Test Chi/Adult | .011 | 26 | -.114 | 10 | -.213 | 11 | .393 | 5 |
| Sentence Repetition | .582 | 124 | .648 | 50 | .459 | 52 | .444 | 22 |
| Lateral Dominance | .869 | 105 | .752 | 42 | .918 | 41 | .895 | 22 |
| Handedness | .707 | 133 | .559 | 55 | .872 | 52 | .936 | 26 |
| Grip Strength, left hand | .365 | 111 | .528 | 43 | .111 | 45 | .397 | 23 |
| Grip Strength, right hand | .362 | 111 | .660 | 43 | .027 | 45 | .360 | 23 |
| WRAT, Reading | .745 | 80 | .761 | 33 | .814 | 33 | .574 | 14 |
| WRAT, Spelling | .729 | 80 | .784 | 34 | .870 | 32 | .505 | 14 |
| WRAT, Arithmetic | .651 | 80 | .738 | 34 | .572 | 32 | .488 | 14 |
| R-L Orientation | .272 | 97 | .255 | 35 | .336 | 44 | .144 | 18 |
| WISC-R/WAIS-R | | | | | | | | |
|   Information | .679 | 119 | .798 | 48 | .500 | 50 | .612 | 21 |
|   Comprehension | .580 | 113 | .624 | 44 | .570 | 50 | .394 | 19 |
|   Arithmetic | .490 | 120 | .573 | 49 | .458 | 50 | .401 | 21 |
|   Similarities | .617 | 118 | .603 | 48 | .552 | 50 | .713 | 21 |
|   Vocabulary | .641 | 116 | .753 | 46 | .499 | 50 | .596 | 20 |
|   Digit Span | .657 | 110 | .649 | 41 | .744 | 48 | .230 | 21 |
|   Picture Completion | .549 | 118 | .627 | 47 | .334 | 50 | .559 | 21 |
|   Picture Arrangement | .517 | 109 | .512 | 42 | .455 | 46 | .362 | 21 |
|   Block Design | .626 | 120 | .604 | 48 | .690 | 51 | .485 | 21 |
|   Object Assembly | .583 | 90 | .597 | 34 | .569 | 38 | .463 | 18 |
|   Coding | .502 | 115 | .429 | 42 | .639 | 51 | .285 | 22 |
| VIQ | .788 | 124 | .860 | 48 | .719 | 55 | .694 | 21 |
| PIQ | .726 | 121 | .779 | 45 | .690 | 55 | .512 | 21 |
| FSIQ | .794 | 118 | .829 | 44 | .777 | 54 | .649 | 20 |

In general, correlation coefficients were high and significant. The highest stability was found for tests of lateral dominance, followed by IQ tests, academic achievement, handedness, and sentence repetition. The coefficients were relatively poor on the Category Test, grip strength, and right-left orientation. This is probably due to the change from the intermediate to the adult version of the Category Test, and, in the case of right-left orientation, to near-perfect scores at the adult age (Benton et al. 1983). Although no consistent pattern of the magnitude of correlations across the three LD groups emerged, there was a trend for group-1 subjects to show the highest correlations, the group-2 subjects to show somewhat lower correlations, and group-3 subjects to have relatively low correlations. Hence, it may be concluded that tests in group 3 are the least stable in this battery of tests. Table 23-2 shows the correlations for IQ-matched groups, which are not substantially different from those shown on Table 23-1.

*Table 23-2: Correlation Coefficients for Corresponding Test*
*Given at a Mean Age of 10 and 25 Years in LD Subject Groups*
*Matched for IQ*

| Test | All Ss | *n* | BD | *n* | MBD | *n* | LD | *n* |
|---|---|---|---|---|---|---|---|---|
| Category Test | .484 | 57 | .601 | 20 | .501 | 29 | .828 | 4 |
| Sentence Repetition | .214 | 97 | .600 | 30 | .488 | 45 | .206 | 22 |
| Lateral Dominance | .901 | 83 | .825 | 25 | .920 | 37 | .894 | 21 |
| Handedness | .827 | 99 | .715 | 31 | .862 | 44 | .935 | 24 |
| Grip Strength, left hand | .310 | 84 | .201 | 24 | .086 | 38 | .400 | 22 |
| Grip Strength, right hand | .342 | 84 | .235 | 24 | .401 | 38 | .355 | 22 |
| WRAT, Reading | .750 | 59 | .779 | 17 | .807 | 29 | .553 | 13 |
| WRAT, Spelling | .693 | 59 | .748 | 18 | .849 | 28 | .450 | 13 |
| WRAT, Arithmetic | .592 | 59 | .694 | 18 | .583 | 28 | .485 | 13 |
| Right-Left Orientation | .192 | 79 | .105 | 22 | .312 | 39 | .144 | 18 |
| WISC-R/WAIS-R | | | | | | | | |
|   Information | .585 | 93 | .732 | 29 | .410 | 43 | .612 | 21 |
|   Comprehension | .457 | 90 | .496 | 28 | .454 | 43 | .394 | 19 |
|   Arithmetic | .347 | 93 | .296 | 29 | .383 | 43 | .401 | 21 |
|   Similarities | .566 | 92 | .543 | 29 | .511 | 42 | .713 | 21 |
|   Vocabulary | .590 | 92 | .771 | 29 | .414 | 43 | .596 | 20 |
|   Digit Span | .615 | 86 | .584 | 24 | .745 | 41 | .230 | 21 |
|   Picture Completion | .431 | 89 | .601 | 27 | .267 | 42 | .517 | 20 |
|   Picture Arrangement | .412 | 83 | .372 | 24 | .475 | 39 | .301 | 20 |
|   Block Design | .651 | 91 | .622 | 28 | .723 | 43 | .567 | 20 |
|   Object Assembly | .524 | 67 | .545 | 19 | .541 | 31 | .457 | 17 |
|   Coding | .438 | 89 | .295 | 25 | .620 | 43 | .385 | 21 |
| VIQ | .615 | 105 | .817 | 31 | .670 | 50 | .482 | 24 |
| PIQ | .761 | 104 | .654 | 30 | .637 | 50 | .688 | 24 |
| FS-IQ | .713 | 104 | .737 | 30 | .734 | 60 | .688 | 24 |

The multivariate analysis of each test as a repeated measure revealed significant time effects in several tests. These time effects reflect an increase in score consistent with the sequential acquisition of the measured skill with age. IQ-test measures were slightly lower for time 2 compared to time

120

1 for all three LD groups. This may reflect a true minor reduction in cognitive skills, but more likely must be viewed as the result of the administration of the recently revised WAIS-R with newly standardized norms.

The results may be viewed as an indication of good long-term reliability or as an indication of long-term persistence of neuropsychological deficit as the child matures from middle childhood to adulthood. The correlation coefficients for the three subgroups provide an estimate of the range of reliability in three different samples.

*Table 23-3. Means of Selected Neuropsychological Tests at Time Referral and at Re-Test 15 Years Later*

| Test | BD | MBD | LD | BD | MBD | LD | Group Effect | Time Effect |
|------|----|----|----|----|----|----|------|------|
| | | Time 1 | | | Time 2 | | | |
| R-L Orientation | 20.9 | 21.5 | 22.1 | 27.3 | 27.8 | 28.1 | n.s. | .001 |
| WRAT Reading | 3.6 | 4.1 | 4.2 | 7.3 | 7.4 | 8.0 | n.s. | .001 |
| WRAT Spelling | 3.3 | 3.4 | 4.0 | 6.1 | 5.6 | 6.2 | n.s. | .001 |
| WRAT Arithmetic | 3.0 | 3.4 | 3.9 | 5.1 | 5.0 | 5.5 | n.s. | .001 |
| Category Test | | | | | | | | |
| Int./Adult | 65.7 | 55.4 | 59.7 | 28.7 | 32.4 | 23.3 | n.s. | .001 |
| Lateral Dominance | 11.9 | 10.8 | 11.6 | 11.9 | 10.9 | 11.5 | n.s. | n.s. |
| Sentence | | | | | | | | |
| Repetition | 10.4 | 11.3 | 11.9 | 13.9 | 14.8 | 15.0 | .017 | .001 |
| Category Test | | | | | | | | |
| Child/Adult | 29.8 | 26.1 | 22.8 | 37.3 | 33.8 | 29.6 | n.s. | .05 |
| Handedness | 1.3 | 1.2 | 1.2 | 1.2 | 1.2 | 1.2 | n.s. | .013 |
| Grip Strength, L | 11.1 | 13.4 | 12.0 | 31.9 | 35.0 | 35.3 | n.s. | .001 |
| Grip Strength, R | 12.1 | 14.0 | 13.1 | 35.1 | 35.8 | 38.0 | n.s. | .001 |

Table 23-3 shows the mean values for each test in the three groups both at time 1 and time 2. Even though the difference between the three groups does not reach an acceptable level of significance except on the sentence repetition test, many of the tests show a linear trend with the poorest values (or highest error score) in group 1 and the best values in group 3. The analysis described in Section 20 demonstrated that these test results do contribute to group discrimination if treated in a multivariate manner and together with other results. The tests available both at time 1 and 2 are limited in number and not the best selection from a predictive point of view. These particular tests must be interpreted with caution in decisions about the presence or absence of 'brain damage', since Table 23-3 does not suggest confidence in their validity as individual measures.

In *summary*, this section reports strong stability for a number of neuropsychological tests over a 15-year period. Alternatively, these results can also be viewed as an expression of high trait stability in our participants. Age-related changes were evident for some tests, as expected, but standardized test scores, e.g., IQ-scores remained highly reliable over time. Among the four groups, group 3 showed the lowest stability.

## 24. The Significance of IQ

Because our four groups differed in overall IQ both at initial referral and at Phase II testing, the question must be raised how much of the differences can be attributed to IQ differences alone. While, on the one hand, these IQ differences are expected and meaningful in that LD groups are expected to function at a lower IQ level than controls, and that neurological handicap lowers IQ scores compared to 'minimal' neurological handicap or lack of neurological findings, it can be argued that many of the differences between groups could be the function of IQ alone, and hence need further detailed analysis.

To investigate the validity of this argument, covariance analysis with IQ of all variables provides one answer. If covariance with IQ is insignificant, then the results remain meaningful above and beyond the discrepancy in IQ. Another method of investigating this question more directly is by IQ matching. Matching of all three LD and the control group is difficult because the IQ difference is fairly large. However, the more important question posed in this study is the difference between three LD groups differing in degree of neurological impairment.

For these reasons, matching of the three LD groups for mean and range of IQ was attempted. Group 3 with the highest IQ and the lowest number of subjects was left intact. None of the subjects in group 3 had IQs below 80. To achieve a match in range, subjects with IQs below 80 in Groups 1 and 2 were excluded. A few additional subjects were excluded in the higher IQ ranges to obtain an optimal match. It should be noted that exclusion of subjects was based on IQ scores and on sequential order of occurrence of a subject in the file (presumably random); any other information about these subjects was not considered.

The three IQ matched LD groups were: (1) 32 subjects in Group 1 with a mean IQ of 96.91, (2) 50 subjects in Group 2 with a mean IQ of 97.00, (3) 24 subjects in Group 3 with a mean IQ of 97.00. Differences between groups on individual IQ-subtests after IQ matching were minimal and insignificant, except for the coding subtest (means 7.19, 8.14, and 9.57 respectively).

In the body of this report, several analyses repeated with IQ-matched LD groups have been reported. All these analyses refer to the groups as described above. In general, IQ matching changed the results of formal testing slightly and in a few instances, differences between the three LD groups were no longer significant. On the other hand, many of the differences between groups on other variables (social, educational, health) remained unchanged and in a few cases became even more pronounced in spite of the fact that reducing the $n$ in our groups inevitably leads to loss of statistical power in the analyses.

A final attempt force-matched all four groups (i.e.,including the control group) on FS-IQ scores by deleting subjects at the low or high end of the IQ distribution until comparable means and ranges were achieved. The means and ranges were: Group 1: 95.96 (range 85-121, $n=23$), Group 2: 95.74 (range 84-125, $n=35$), Group 3: 96.22 (range 84-111, $n=18$), Group 4: 98.07 (range 79-105, $n=14$). This, of course, severely reduces the number of subjects available for group comparisons. A number of analyses of the employment variables at Phases I and II were repeated. For the Phase I data, the trend remained unchanged between groups, although statistical significance was not reached with the small number of subjects (e.g., 'Did you have difficulties finding a job'? Group means: 46, 36, 14, and 4.5%, chi-square $= 7.10$, $p= .06$. Age when first job was started? Group means: 14.7, 14.1, 14.4, 13.1, $F= .998$, $p < .039$). For the Phase II data, similar results were obtained as in the main analyses, but again failed to obtain statistical significance with the lower number of subjects (e.g., percent of subjects employed on a permanent rather than a part-time basis ( 43.5, 73, 61, 79 , chi-square$= 6.62$, $p< .08$). Strikingly, the sex difference in salary on the longest held job (males \$ 1469, females \$ 1146) and the highest monthly salary received during the past 5 years (males \$ 1909, females \$ 1282) remained highly significant even with the small sample.

In *summary*, the three LD groups showed differences in mean IQ-scores even after deletion of participants with an IQ of less than 70. The more neurological impairment, the lower was the group IQ. This led to reanalyses of the results reported in several sections with IQ-matched LD groups, as well as to analysis of covariance. This section describes the matching procedure, as well as a force-matching of the three LD groups with the control group on FS-IQ. The basic trends of the results reported throughout this monograph did not change after IQ-matching although in some instances statistical significance was lost, both for Phase I and Phase II data.

### 25. Comparison between Parents' and Student's Responses

During the Phase I follow-up two essentially identical interviews were carried out independently, one with the participant (former client) and one with one or both of his/her parents. The two sources can be compared in order to obtain reliability estimates for the responses to each question. More importantly, the two respondents may produce genuine differences in opinion on many questions since parts of the interview did not call for facts alone, but for opinions about adjustment, satisfaction, etc. It would be of specific interest to see which of the two respondents would take a more optimistic view of the participants' progress through the years, and whether such differences are consistent across the four groups.

The method of analysis for this information was a 2 source levels (students/parents) by 4 group levels (groups 1 through 4) analysis of variance as shown in Table 25-1. In this illustration, the question was 'Do you think other people see you as different?', followed by the question 'Who sees you as different?'. The answers were coded as ranging from 'everyone, everywhere' through 'Mom, Dad, brothers, sisters, others at home, classmates, teachers, co-workers' to 'I'm not sure who' and 'others'. For this analysis the sum of all possible choices was calculated, i.e.,the sum of all people who were mentioned as seeing the participant as different. However, since the answer 'everyone' reflected the opinion of being viewed as different in many situations and by many people, this answer was assigned 5 points rather than 1 as an arbitrary weight; the results remained significant even without such weighting , i.e., if 'everyone' was coded as '1'.

*Table 25-1: Number of People Who View Participant as 'Different' from Others as Reported by Parents and Participants for the Four Groups and Covariance with Age and IQ Score*

| Means | BD | SBD | LD | C |
|---|---|---|---|---|
| students | 1.41 | 1.40 | 0.67 | 0.77 |
| parents | 3.03 | 2.11 | 1.44 | 0.43 |
| both | 2.22 | 1.76 | 1.05 | 0.60 |
| Main effects | $F$ | $p$ | | |
| Group | 5.47 | .005 | | |
| Parent/Student | 5.43 | .0011 | | |
| Interaction | 0.65 | ns | | |
| Regression | | | | |
| Age | .03 | | | |
| IQ | -.023 | | | |
| Covariates | | | | |
| Age | 0.34 | ns | | |
| IQ | 8.59 | .004 | | |

The table shows that for the group 1 an average of more than two people were mentioned who viewed the client as different; however, parents indicated an average of 3 while the clients mentioned only an average of 1.4 people. The figures are lower for groups 2 and 3, but again parents felt that more people saw their child as different than the participants themselves. This trend is reversed for the control group: not only was there only a small group who viewed themselves as different, but students rather than parents reported more often that this was the case. The analysis also included covariance with age and IQ at the time of referral. This part of the analysis shows that age does not significantly affect the results, but that being viewed as 'different' tends to increase as IQ decreases.

Similar analyses have been included in most of the previously reported results. Somewhat similar results to the ones described above were found for the question whether the participant was 'feeling happy' and 'are you usually satisfied with your life now?'. No differences between parent and student interview were observed on the reported plans for next year and plans for the more distant future. It would seem that the differences between parent and student interview do not occur when tangible facts (i.e.,plans for next year) are asked for. This holds generally true for most parts of the interview.

Two possible explanations offer themselves for the observed differences between parent and student responses to questions concerning subjective feelings: (a) students are defensive about their feelings and tend to describe themselves in more optimistic terms than their parents; (b) parents are overly concerned, especially for our more seriously impaired participants, have perhaps assumed an overprotective attitude, and tend to overestimate the amount of dissatisfaction and alienation. That these differences reverse themselves on some questions for the control group and the fact that our subjects were generally open and cooperative in their attitude during the interview suggests that perhaps the second explanation is more appropriate. However, both explanations must be considered.

Further differences between parent and participant responses were found in parts of the interview related to the earlier development of our clients. For example, behaviour problems before the time of referral were reported significantly more often by parents than by participants. This may reflect the fact that the participants simply do not remember that part of their lives accurately enough; for the period following the referral and up to the Phase I interview the differences between parent and subject interview are no longer significant. This explanation is supported by responses to the question: 'How well do you recall that period of your life?', i.e.,before the referral at age 8-12; 70 to 88% of groups 2, 3, and 4 answered 'very well', but only 49% of group 1 did so (a significant difference). This interpretation may also apply to the significant difference between parent and participant responses to the question whether they ever had a problem which the parent and/or teacher did not understand.

Similar results without significant interactions were found for other adjustment and health-related questions: Parents reported health problems and seizures prior to the time of referral more frequently; parents reported more often the need for drug treatment prior to the referral age than the students; parents reported that their son/daughter was getting along better with others than reported by the participants themselves;

parents gave more reasons for a change in the general health of their child than did the participants. On the other hand, subjects reported that they got along better with teachers, siblings, father and mother than what was reported by the parents; the participants also described the relationship within the family as poorer than the parents did. Participants also reported more often the use of alcohol and drugs than their parents.

The participants reported that they had more jobs than their parents said, and that they had started their first job earlier; they recorded less enjoyment of the work than parents.

Subjects also admitted more often that they had come to the attention of the police. They reported a larger number of close friends and more often friends of the opposite sex than parents; they reported fewer phone calls from friends. The participants also reported more accidents since the time of referral than parents.

In comparison with the participants, the parents more often answered yes to the question whether there was something the interviewee wanted to see changed in his/her life; parents also reported more specific incidences which they felt had hindered or helped their child in his/her learning. Finally, parents reported helping more often with homework, and that awards in school were less common.

On all other questions no significant differences between parents' and students' responses were found. In general, the comparison of parent and student interview seems to indicate good reliability of responses to more factual questions. The differences between the two interviews described above relate to questions calling for an opinion or judgement and to some factual questions where parents may not be aware of the actual situation (e.g., alcohol, drug use, coming to the attention of the police), and where participants probably provided a more realistic or honest response. Other questions which produced differences between the two sources of information concerned interpersonal relations and seem to reflect a more optimistic view on the part of the subjects and/or overconcern or a more pessimistic attitude on the part of the parents.

In *summary*, the comparison between parents' and participants' responses to the age-18 interview showed good agreement on factual questions. On questions concerning delinquency, drug and alcohol use, participants responded more often with 'yes' than parents. On questions calling for an opinion about getting along with others, outlook on life, life satisfaction and similar matters the parents showed a more negative response pattern than the subjects in our study, perhaps suggesting an overprotective attitude of parents at that time.

## 26. The Effect of Treatment on Outcome

One of the weaknesses of this study was that the investigators worked with 'natural' groups coming from many different schools and districts, and hence had no control over the treatment available to the participants except for recommendations made to the referring physician and to the school after the initial assessment. As described in section 12, the assistance was extremely variable although adequate in terms of the resources available.

An attempt was made to list all intervention received by each participant carefully during the follow-up interviews. This formed the basis of a first analysis aimed at the relationship between intervention and outcome. The following educational intervention variables were selected: need for special help in school, summer school, counselling, help at home, special class, special instruction in school, school learning assistance teacher, private tutoring, other special help. The variables were continuous, i.e.,each variable was scored as the number of school grades during which such intervention occurred, and submitted to a principal component analysis. The analysis yielded four significant factors with Eigenvalues greater than 1, accounting for 60% of the variance. Since the fourth factor had major loadings only on 'other special help', it was treated as a residual and omitted (together with the variable itself) from further consideration (Table 26-1).

*Table 26-1: Three Intervention Factors*

| Factor | 1 | 2 | 3 |
|---|---|---|---|
| help in school | 83 | 10 | -15 |
| summer school | 04 | 64 | 18 |
| counselling | 18 | 54 | -39 |
| home help | 74 | 15 | 13 |
| special class | 74 | -15 | -70 |
| special instruction | 01 | 71 | 05 |
| learning assistance teacher | 29 | 00 | 66 |
| private tutoring | 48 | -24 | 21 |

While the first factor appears to represent a more general educational intervention factor including attendence in special class, the second factor consists mainly of counselling, special instruction, and summer school, i.e.,a less invasive type of intervention, negatively related to special class and tutoring. The third factor is a 'special class' factor with inverted loadings for other forms of intervention.

Similarly, some of the more critical outcome variables were factor analyzed in an attempt to relate the two sets of variables. A principal

127

component analysis included the following outcome variables: Scores on achievement tests, WAIS-R vocabulary, arithmetic, highest school grade completed, answers to the questions: 'Do you still have this learning problem now?', 'Did you have difficulty finding a job?', 'Are you working now?', degree programs completed, full-time employment, permanent employment, salary, source of income, 'Do you like to read?', 'Do you read much?', 'Do you see yourself as different from others?', number of jobs held, scores on memory passages, visual reproduction, paired-associate learning, delayed memory of the Wechsler Memory Test, WAIS-R digit span, type of current job, duration of school, vocational school or college attendence during the last five years at Phase II interview. The analysis resulted in seven meaningful factors (Table 26-2).

*Table 26-2: Principal Component Factors of Outcome Variables*

| Factors<br>Variables | 1 | 2 | 3 | 4 | 5 | 6 | 7 |
|---|---|---|---|---|---|---|---|
| WRAT Reading | 79 | 12 | 05 | 07 | -09 | 32 | 15 |
| WRAT Spelling | 82 | -03 | 12 | 00 | -23 | 17 | 02 |
| WRAT Arithmetic | 67 | 38 | 19 | -02 | 35 | -03 | -10 |
| PIAT Reading Comp. | 52 | 44 | 09 | 01 | 05 | 45 | 26 |
| WAIS Arithmetic | 69 | 36 | 18 | -02 | 29 | -01 | -09 |
| WAIS Vocabulary | 46 | 50 | 27 | -06 | 04 | 35 | 19 |
| WAIS Comprehension | 30 | 46 | 33 | -05 | 28 | 28 | 21 |
| Grades Completed | 37 | 17 | 47 | 05 | -03 | -13 | 12 |
| Still a Problem | 70 | -04 | 12 | 11 | 15 | -08 | 22 |
| Diff. Jobfinding | 14 | -41 | -12 | -18 | -17 | 14 | -11 |
| Degrees, Diplomas | 01 | 04 | 71 | 14 | 06 | 01 | 06 |
| Working now | -05 | 00 | 15 | 82 | 13 | 00 | -17 |
| Full-time Work | -06 | 01 | 09 | 00 | 06 | 00 | 75 |
| Permanent Employment | -01 | -13 | -22 | 56 | 19 | 03 | 50 |
| Salary | -06 | -04 | 03 | 39 | 70 | 07 | -09 |
| Source of Income | 03 | 00 | 15 | 86 | 06 | -01 | 13 |
| Likes to Read | 07 | 11 | 09 | 02 | 03 | 83 | -13 |
| Reads much | 26 | 24 | 07 | -01 | -01 | 77 | 12 |
| Number of Jobs | 03 | 09 | 60 | 15 | 02 | 07 | -17 |
| Memory Passages | 18 | 75 | 22 | -07 | 12 | 23 | -16 |
| Visual Reproduction | 09 | 44 | -08 | -01 | 51 | -05 | 34 |
| Paired Ass. Learng. | 25 | 72 | -12 | 10 | -25 | 09 | -01 |
| Delayed Memory | 05 | 80 | 19 | -05 | 05 | 12 | 01 |
| Jobtype | -07 | 03 | 09 | 07 | 80 | 01 | 15 |
| School last 5 years | 10 | 16 | 75 | -03 | 04 | 17 | 07 |

Factor 1 appears to be mainly an achievement test factor; factor 2, a verbal performance factor; factor 3 is best represented by postsecondary school attendance and employment; factor 4 is a general employment factor; factor 5 represents level of employment and salary, factor 6, current reading interests; and factor 7, full-time and permanent aspects of employment. Four variables were deleted from the list since they were represented by residual factors only.

In a canonical analysis comparing the set of educational treatment variables with the set of outcome variables described above, only the first canonical correlation was significant ($r = .755, p < .01$). This canonical correlation drew its main treatment effect from 'attendence in special class', and related mainly to the first factor of the outcome variables, i.e.,the full set of achievement test scores (negative loadings). The relationship expressed in this canonical correlation is obvious: participants who had attended special classes in school had poor achievement test results; most other variables of the outcome set were also negatively related to the first treatment factor, although with lower first factor loadings.

Other canonical correlations in this analysis, although not statistically significant, point out some other possible relationships between intervention and outcome: canonical correlation 2 ($r = .676, p < .20$) between private tutoring and holding a permanent job suggests that motivation and possibly parental influence contribute to a more positive outcome. The remainder of the canonical correlations did not yield any significant relationships nor did they carry exceptionally high loadings suitable for interpretation.

In general, the exploration of the intervention-outcome dimension was disappointing. Whether one can describe the result as a 'lack' of intervention effects (except for the first canonical correlation), i.e.,failure of intervention to change the outcome, or whether this is due to the high variability of our participants in terms of intervention approaches, remains to be resolved in other studies specifically aimed at intervention effects.

In *summary*, the educational and other treatment variables were factor analyzed. Only the variables of the first factor, representing general treatment and special class placement, showed a significant relation to outcome, i.e., the achievement test variables at age 25 (the first outcome factor). Private tutoring during the school years was also related to holding a permanent job at age 25; this canonical correlation was not significant, but points to a possible relationship between occupational outcome and motivation and parental influence.

# C. SUMMARY AND CONCLUSIONS

Phase I

Two hundred and three children and their parents were interviewed an average of 9 (between 4 and 12) years after their first initial referral and assessment for LD at the University of Victoria Neuropsychology Clinic. The sample was broken down into three groups according to the degree of neurological impairment (definite impairment = group 1, suggested impairment = group 2, learning disability without clinically demonstrated neurological impairment = group 3). A control group of 52 youngsters (group 4) matched for age, sex, and socioeconomic status, and selected from regional secondary school records, were also interviewed. The average age in all four groups was 19 years. The interview covered a wide range of issues: school experience and attitudes (success/failure, highest grade achieved, special instruction, awards, special competence or problems), employment history, health (general health, illness, seizures, accidents, drugs), family characteristics and relationships, other personal relations (marriage, dating, friends), behaviour problems, involvement with the police, offenses, penalties resulting, as well as a behaviour rating scale filled in by the parents, and a personality questionnaire (Bell 1962) completed by the participants. The results of Phase I have been reported in a number of papers (Denbigh 1979; Hern 1979; Hern & Spreen, in press; Peter & Spreen 1979; Spreen 1978a, 1981, 1982, 1983a, b; Spreen & Lawriw 1980).

Perhaps the most important finding of the Phase I follow-up was that, on a majority of outcome variables, a definite and significant difference was found between the four groups. Usually, this difference was present in a linear fashion, i.e., LD children without neurological impairment (group 3) fared worse than the control group (group 4); children with evidence of minimal or questionable brain dysfunction (group 2) showed poorer outcome than those without neurological impairment, and the definitely brain-damaged group (group 1) showed the poorest outcome of all four groups. In all areas of long-term adjustment and outcome (educational, social, personal, occupational) the presence of neurological handicap was related to poorer achievement and adjustment even though these groups differed only slightly in general intelligence at the time of the original referral several years ago, and mentally retarded subjects were excluded from the comparisons.

131

In the area of academic achievement it was found that the three LD groups were inferior to the control group in all areas including art, industrial education, as well as academic subjects, and in attitudes towards school, but no differences were found in physical education or in involvement with extracurricular activities. Few reliable differences in academic achievement were found between groups of LD children with different degrees of neurological involvement. A strikingly low rate of educational counselling received in all four groups was noted. The analysis of the behaviour rating scale and the personality questionnaire revealed consistent significant relationships between an earlier diagnosis of neurological impairment and behavioural deviance at the time of the follow-up, even when confounding variables such as age, sex, and intelligence were taken into account (Peter & Spreen 1979). All LD groups reported a greater number of indications of emotional maladjustment and more antisocial behaviour than the control group. Surprisingly, females were found to have more social and personality problems than males. Health adjustment was more impaired in females than in males, which may account for the more severe social difficulties. In addition, the number of reported central nervous system illnesses, seizures, and problems of the mother during pregnancy and birth, decreased as the level of neurological impairment decreased (Hern & Spreen, in press). General health and the number of accidents sustained were not significantly different in the presence of a LD or neurologic dysfunction. This latter finding is somewhat contradictory to previous research (Wender 1971; Kinsbourne 1973) which claimed that such children are 'accident prone'. Considering the relationship between learning disorders and delinquency, Spreen (1981) found no increase in the number of encounters with the police or the number of offenses committed by LD youngsters compared to controls. This finding stands in contrast to some results from retrospective studies (e.g. Berman 1978a, b) in which a pronounced association between LD and delinquency was reported.

Control group children also attended school longer, had slightly higher salaries, and were less likely to have received psychological and psychiatric counselling than learning handicapped children.

The Phase I findings make some contribution to the clarification of the controversial term 'minimal brain dysfunction'. The concept is a weak one in that it often refers to the mere inference of brain dysfunction from behavioural observations and tests or from 'soft neurological signs' which may be merely transient, maturational, or hard to elicit. Our study used the concept in clearly defined operational terms, based on a neurological examination rather than on inference from other sources. Stated in this form, children falling into this category could then be contrasted with those with 'hard' evidence of neurological impairment and those without such signs. Our study was the first to attempt this contrast, and the results clearly indicate that children with 'minimal brain dysfunction' show

132

poorer outcome than those without such evidence, but better outcome than those with definite neurological impairment. This result was not anticipated when the study was designed, but seems to confirm clearly that evidence of minimal brain dysfunction (defined in these operational terms) has a significant impact on the future development of the child. One restriction should be stated, however : minimal brain dysfunction was only assessed by a neurological examination between the age of 8 and 12 years. Hence our results cannot necessarily be generalized to children in whom such evidence is demonstrated at an earlier age, although it is likely that in most of our participants the neurological deficit was congenital.

The results have shown considerable social and economic implications: not only do these youngsters suffer through a miserable and usually shortened school career, live a discouraging social life, full of disappointments and failures, they also have fewer chances for adequate employment and advanced training.

Our two separate interviews (with the participants and their parents) indicated that parents are well aware of the difficulties encountered by their children. On questions concerning factual information, the two interviews showed good agreement, with the exception of the areas of encounters with the police, alcohol and drug use, where parents usually reported fewer instances than the clients themselves (probably because the parents were not aware of the full extent of such behaviour). On the other hand, parents tended to report much more serious effects on the personal well-being, happiness, and social interaction of their children, i.e., they took a more pessimistic view than the clients reported. This may reflect an over-protective attitude on the part of the parent obtaining into early adulthood since our control group did not show this discrepancy between client and parent responses. It was also apparent that LD children remember health-related and behaviour problems before the age of 8 to 12 less well than their parents and less well than control subjects; it would appear that their childhood memories were not as clear as those of other children.

Our former clients ranged in age from 13 to 25 years. As age increased, all of our subjects tended to have firmer plans for the future and better occupational adjustment. However, with increasing degree of neurological impairment, our clients had more difficulty in finding a job, finding more than temporary employment, and had less earnings; with increasing age, our clients also indicated increasingly negative memories about their school experiences.

Phase II

A second follow-up was conducted approximately 6½ years later when our participants were in their mid-twenties. As in the Phase I study, it was obvious that former LD children were at a definite disadvantage in many areas during their young adult years. Some of the differences between our LD subjects and controls became somewhat attenuated. However, health problems, especially seizures, persisted. Learning problems reflected in academic achievement tests were clearly not overcome, but put LD youngsters at a disadvantage in finding advanced education and vocational opportunities. Job types and average income levels were lower. Personal adjustment is strained from childhood on, and while some of our subjects showed less turmoil in their personal relations and emotional adjustment than at the Phase I interview, such problems are still much more prevalent than in our control subject population.

The role of neurological impairment in long-term outcome was a key point of interest in this study. A majority of our findings support the contention that the presence of neurological findings in LD children is related to poorer outcome, even if overall IQ level is deliberately matched between LD groups. The group-2 subjects with 'minimal' neurological findings follow this trend. As defined in our study, such minimal signs were associated with poorer outcome not as severe as in the 'definite brain damage' group, but more serious than in the LD group without neurological findings. Our study further showed that most of the so-called 'minimal' findings do not disappear with the maturation of the individual, but persist into adulthood and that some of these signs actually increase in frequency. This is a new finding which is contrary to the notion that such signs are maturational in nature and would disappear with time. In the absence of other long-term studies of this topic, this result should be treated with caution, and requires replication.

In addition to the update interview covering the years between Phase I and II of the follow-up, the Phase II recall also included the administration of a large number of objective tests, a neurological reexamination and a personality test. Since these were administered by examiners blind to the previous neurological status, the Phase I information and the Phase II update interview, and since cooperation during these examinations was, on the whole, very good, the data from these examinations represent, at least in part, objective confirmation of the results based on interviews.

On reexamination, neurological impairment continued to persist in a majority of our participants. While some of the "hard signs" were less frequent in the neurologically handicapped group, the groups which had no such signs on intake did show a surprising number of these signs on adult examination."Soft" signs persisted in the majority of the neurologically impaired groups, but also appeared for the first time on reexamination of the LD group which was without neurological findings at intake, but only in a small number of control group subjects. This must be interpreted as an indication that most "soft" neurological signs are not maturational inconsistencies or due to inattention, but represent a persistent , probably life-long impairment. In particular, neurological signs in

134

the sensory and speech domain showed a high degree of persistence. The significance of the neurological findings for the long-term outcome of LD has, of course, been the main focus of this report. Relating the neurological findings to school achievement, a canonical analysis showed a strong relationship between overall achievement and motor integrity, one major factor of the neurological examination.

Intelligence test scores as well as the scores of other tests repeated at age 25 showed a very high degree of long-term reliability when age 10 and age 25 tests were compared. IQ-score differences among the three LD groups and between LD and control groups still persisted, and the effect of these differences on other test results was considered by covariance analysis and by forced group matching for IQ. Even after matching, many of our group differences in most areas of the investigation persisted.

Left-handedness and ambilaterality were significantly higher in our LD groups compared to the control group. However, no significant increase in left-handedness or ambilaterality with degree of neurological impairment was found. Handedness remained consistent from intake to adult age. The decreased incidence of dexterity in this LD population can be interpreted as consistent with the increase in neurological dysfunction suggested by the neurological examination.

On several other tests, especially those of concentration and memory, the LD groups showed inferior performance compared to controls, frequently following the pattern of linear decrease with increasing neurological findings, even after matching for IQ. The same result also obtained for measures of motor dexterity (pegboard), finger localization, and right-left orientation.

In an analysis of personality characteristics behaviour ratings by parents, by interviewers and some self-report statements were factor analyzed and three major factors extracted from this information: (1) impulsivity/negativity, (2) temper/fighting, (3) hyperactivity/behaviour problems. LD subjects ranked on the negative end of these scales more frequently, and groups 1 and 2 were more often rated as "taciturn, quiet, no spontaneous conservation" compared to group 3 and controls who were more loquacious. Other differences between LD groups and controls were found for "seriousness" and "appropriateness".

The MMPI as a major measure of personal adjustment showed significant group differences even after elimination of poor readers and low IQ subjects. All validity and clinical scales except Hy ('hysteria'), Mf ('masculinity/femininity'), and Ma ('mania') showed elevated scores for the LD groups. In addition, three depression subscales, the Hy1 (Denial of Social Anxiety), Pd4A (Social Alienation), Sc2B (Lack of Ego Mastery), and the Ego Strength scales all showed significantly deviant scores for the LD groups. The LD groups generally differed in linear fashion with the most abnormal scores in group 1 and the least abnormal in group 3, although the differences between groups are not statistically significant. It was noted that elevations usually were not in the clinically abnormal ($T$ score $> 70$) range. The percentage of abnormal scores in each group suggested, however, that, when clinically elevated scores do occur, they are usually found in groups 1 and 2.

Predictive validity of the intake test results for outcome at age 18 and 25 was investigated by canonical analysis. A highly significant canonical correlation suggested that measures of verbal intelligence and academic achievement at intake are strongly related to outcome, especially as measured by adjustment inventory scores. The section also describes an analysis of the contribution of socio-economic status of the parents to adult outcome. A distinct and significant contribution was found, accounting for 28% of the variance (O'Connor & Spreen 1986).

Subtypes of LD were investigated by empirical (hierarchical) grouping analysis. Eight clusters were found, two of which were severity-specific (near-normal and severely impaired); one cluster represented specific arithmetic disability, and one specific reading disability; one additional cluster was seen mainly as visuo-perceptual deficit, and the other as a primary language-related deficit.

A replication of the cluster analysis with additional subjects showed nine clusters with the specific reading disability divided into a graphomotor and a language-related subtype. Split-half validation was successful.

At adult age, nine clusters were found, but strikingly the language-related cluster was absent. Correspondence between membership in childhood and adult clusters was poor. Subjects who were in the language-related cluster in childhood tended to be found in the severely impaired group as adults.

A detailed analysis of the hyperactivity/attention deficit complex in our population suggested a moderate relationship between hyperactivity and membership in the four groups of subjects (Spreen 1986). Grouping our participants into four activity-level groups showed a mild relationship with neurological findings only in males, but not in the groups overall. Subjects with high activity level on ratings tended to work in more "active" jobtypes at age 18, but this difference was no longer found at age 25. There was a significant relationship between hyperactivity and and poorer outcome on jobs and employment.

While our results in general show persistence of LD and poor outcome in many areas of personal, social, occupational, and health adjustment as well as persistently poorer test scores compared to our control subjects, it should be remembered that these differences are statistical averages which do not clearly express the range of variability across our former LD clients, nor do they fully express the personal experience and suffering which some of them experienced. We found some of our former clients in group homes, even in prison and in a mental hospital, but others lived in comfortable

136

homes of their own and with apparent full adjustment in their community. During the interviews, however, many of our participants relived the years since their first referral to our laboratory, and often expressed their frustration, anger, and depression in forms that cannot be documented in questionnaires or submitted to statistical analysis. We will attempt to describe some of these personal experiences in narrative form at another time.

# D. Appendices

## 1. List of Tests and Other Measurements (Abbreviation in Brackets)

Minnesota Multiphasic Personality Inventory (MMPI)
Rating for Follow-Up Interview Behaviour and Appearance
   a) interviewer    b)examiner
Wechsler Memory Scale, Form I
Wide Range Achievement Test (WRAT)
   a) Reading (WRAT-R)    b) Spelling (WRAT-S)    c) Arithmetic
(WRAT-A)
Lateral Dominance Examination
Grip Strength (Dynamometer)
Finger Localization
Right-Left Orientation (R-L Or)
   a) Standard Form (Benton)    b) Extended Form (Culver)
Wechsler Adult Intelligence Scale - Revised (WAIS-R)
   Arithmetic Subtest (WAIS A)
   Vocabulary Subtest (Vocab)
   Similarities Subtest (Simi)
   Digit Symbol Subtest (Symbol)
Crossing Out Task (Bourdon Test)
Audiogram
Balanced Dichotic Listening Test (DL)
Sentence Repetition Test (Sent.Rep.)
Adult Halstead Category Test, Victoria Revision (Categ.)
Word Fluency Test (WF)
Purdue Pegboard Test
   Both Hands (Purd.B)
   Assembly (Purd.A)
Peabody Individual Achievement Test: Reading Comprehension (PIAT-
C)

## 2. Structured Interview Schedule (Phase I)*

   1. Subject identification number

---

* The parent interview schedule was identical except that she/he was substituted
for you in each question. Coding information has been omitted for most of the
interview.

2. Interviewer
3. Date of interview
4. Sequence of interview for interviewer that day
5. Location of interview

*Family Constellation*

6. How old are you?
7. When were you born?
8. Are you left- or right-handed?
9. Have you always been -handed?
10. Have you ever had any other parents in addition to your natural parents?
11. Who else has been a parent to you?
12. What was the reason?
13. Were you placed out of the home at that time?
14. How old were you?
15. (If school age that year) What grade were you in? Do you feel your school performance changed for better or for worse as a result of what happened then?
16. Have you ever lost a/another parent?
17. Have your parents ever divorced or separated while you were living with them?
18. Are both of your natural parents alive?
19. How many mothers have you had in total?
20. How many fathers have you had in total?
21. Are you living at home (with parents) now?
22. Are you living on your own now?
23. How old were you when you left home the first time?
24. Have you ever lived completely away from parents for any length of time?
25. If yes, how old were you then?
26. If yes, in what school grade were you then?
27. If yes, why did you live away from them?
28. How many months were you away?
29. Did living away from your parents affect you either for better or for worse?
30. How many other people are living with you today?
31. Were you a twin birth?
32. Were you the first born to your mother? (birthrank)
33. Can you name all the other children who live/d at home with you? (sex, age, for how long, relationship)
34. Name all other people who live/d with you (for how long, relationship, handedness)

35. Do you have any brothers or sisters other than the ones who have lived with you? (or half-siblings)
36. How many brothers do you have in all?
37. How many sisters do you have in all?
38. Has any adult in the family ever had any difficulty learning to read or write or speak? (code with list of persons from questions above)

*School Experience*

39. Did you attend preschool (incl. nursery-, play-school, kindergarten, etc.)
40. How old were you when you started preschool?
41. How long did you attend?
42. How old were you when you started school?
43. In which grade did you begin?
44. What school were you in then?
45. Did you go to any other school that year?
46. What grade did you attend the next year? (code for all years and all schools)
47. Are you still attending school?
48. Did you pass the last grade you attended school?
49. Did you ever need special help at school?
50. Were you ever in a special class?
51. Did you ever receive special instruction or special coursework?
52. Did you ever have a learning assistance teacher?
53. Did you ever receive private tutoring or private instruction in school subjects? (code information from this and previous questions for all grades and years attended, separate remedial and advanced instruction)
54. Have you ever attended summer school? (code grade and type of instruction)
55. Which subjects have given you the most trouble?
56. Has anyone in your family regularly helped you with your home work?
57. In general, how did you like school?
58. Did you always feel pretty much the same way? (Code grades liked and not liked)
59. Is there anything in particular that you liked or disliked about school?
60. Were you ever expelled or suspended from school? (age, grade, reason for and length of time)
61. Have you ever received any honours? (cups, prizes, ribbons, certificates or other awards)
62. Was it common practice in all the schools you attended for awards to be granted?

63. Have you ever been nominated or elected officer of a school class, club or of any other organization?
64. Have you ever taken any academic courses at college and/or university?
65. Did you complete a particular program there?
66. Have you ever taken any courses at a trade school or a technical school?
67. How involved have you been in school activities? (code type, time spent, rank order)
68. Altogether, about how many hours a week - outside of regular school hours - did you usually spend on these activities?
69. Did anything ever prevent you from participating in school activities as much as you would have liked to?

*Job and Employment*

70. Have you ever been employed?
71. How many jobs have you had altogether?
72. How old were you when you were first employed?
73. Are you working now?
74. Were you in school when you got this job?
75. What is your job? (code jobtype)
76. Was/Is it full-time?
77. Was/Is it temporary or probably permanent?
78. Is it the kind of job you enjoy doing?
79. Does the job require the best of your abilities?
80. How long have you worked there?
81. What was/is your approximate highest salary per month?
82. Are you poorly paid?
83. Have you ever looked for a job?
84. Have you had any particular difficulty finding a job?
85. What income do you live on?
86. How is your father employed?
87. How is your mother employed?
88. Did/Do you jobs at home or for neighbors or friends?
89. How do you like doing these jobs?
90. When these jobs are to be done, do you think you can be relied upon to do these jobs and do them well?

*Problem and Treatment*

91. The records show that you came to this laboratory for testing in 19-- (You have not been tested here before) Is this correct?
92. How old were you then?
93. Do you remember that time of your life fairly well? For instance, can

you remember what grade you were in, who your teachers were, your classmates, etc.?

94. Can you remember any specific problem you had at that time       years ago that made it difficult for you at adjust to school or at home? Can you remember what specific problem brought you to our laboratory, or any other problems?

95. Up until you were       years old, had you had any health problems (code all health problems with age of onset, length, duration, and all subsequent health problems)?

96. Up until you were       years old, have you had any seizures, fits, convulsions, or epileptic attacks? (Code frequency. duration, age at onset, type of seizure)

97. Have you subsequently had any seizures or fits.etc.?

98. Up until you were       years old, had you had any accidents or injuries? (Code type, age at onset, length of aftereffects)

99. Have you subsequently had any accidents?

100. Up until you were       years old, had you ever had any particular learning problems? (code type, onset, duration)

101. Have you subsequently had any (other) learning problems?

102. Up until you were       years old, had you ever had any behaviour problem? (code type, onset, duration)

103. Have you subsequently had any behaviour problems?

104. Do you feel that you ever had a problem which your parents or teachers did not recognize or understand at that time? (code type, age at onset, duration)

105. Have you ever come to the attention of the police?

106. What were you charged with? (code age and grade)

107. What was the penalty? (code all offenses up to the date of this interview)

108. How is your general health now, compared to the time when you were       years old?

109. Do you know any reason why it has changed?

110. After you were       years old, did your school performance get better or worse?

111. In your last year of school how do you feel you got along with your teachers, better or worse?

112. Did contacting our laboratory at that time help you in any way with your learning difficulties?

113. Do you have any suggestions as to how our services might have been more helpful?

114. Have you ever been to a physician for advice or medical treatment of any of your problems? (code in sequence type of physician,diagnosis, treatment, results, age, grade, and duration)

115. Have you ever been to any other kind of physician or specialist?

116. Have you ever been to a speech and hearing specialist?
117. Have you ever been to a psychiatrist or psychologist?
118. Have you ever had educational counselling?
119. Is there anyone else you have been to for professional advice or medical treatment for any of your problems?
120. Have you taken any medications or prescription drugs up to the time when you were ___ years old?
121. Have you subsequently taken any medication or prescription drugs? (code for drug, purpose, age, length, and effects)
122. Have you ever, accidentally or on purpose, taken a drug not prescribed for you? (other than over-the-counter drugs. meaning prescription or street drugs)
123. Did any of these drugs affect you for better or worse?
124. Do you drink alcoholic beverages?
125. Do you ever have any problems with alcohol?

*Social Adjustment*

126. Have you been married or lived common-law?
127. How old were you when you got married?
128. Were you in school at that time?
129. In general, how would you rate your relationship?
130. Would you say you usually experience a lot of problems, some problems, or no problems at all?
131. Have you ever been separated from your spouse? (code onset of separation, length, frequency)
132. Did you divorce? (age, length of marriage, remarriage)
133. Have you had any children either while married or unmarried?
134. Have you ever dated?
135. Are you dating now?
136. Would you like to date?
137. How do you usually get along with your dates?
138. About how many dates have you had during the last three months?
139. Apart from school/work activities what do you do in your spare time (code all hobbies, sports, group activi- ties etc. by hours per week)
140. Do you have time for friends?
141. In a four-week period, how often would your friends phone you?
142. In the same length of time, how often would you phone your friends?
143. In a four-week period, how often would you visit your friends?
144. In the same length of time, how often would they visit you?
145. How many close friends and how many casual friends do you have?
146. Are you friends equally mixed - both boys and girls - ?
147. In general, are you satisfied with your friends?

148. Can you always find a friend when you need one?
149. In general, how do you feel you get along with others? (specific code for getting along with classmates or co-workers, neighbors, siblings, mother, father)
150. Compared to the time when you were     years old, how often do you now see your mother, father, brothers, and sisters?
151. At present, how do you feel your family gets along together?
152. Is this any different from the way you got along together when you were     years old?
153. Do you think you have reasonable judgement in most matters?
154. Do you ever lose control of your temper?
155. Do you see yourself as different from others of your age?
156. Do you think other people see you as different? (code relationship and number)
157. Compared to when you were     years old, would you say that you, in general, feel happier or less happy now?
158. What experiences would you say were the turning points for better or worse in your life?
159. Are you usually satisfied with the way your life is now?
160. If there is something you would want to change in your life, what would that be?
161. Can you remember any experiences which I did not ask about which you feel helped you with learning, or, one the other hand, held you back?
162. What are your plans for next year?
163. What would you like to be doing after next year?


## 3. Interview and Test Behaviour Rating Scale (Phase I)

*range: 1 to 5 points*

1. Grooming
   1 = overly neat and orderly
   5 = dirty, untidy, disheveled
2. Maturity of behaviour
   1 = 'old' for age, subdued, overly serious
   5 = childish, silly, unable to take situation seriously
3. Manifest Anxiety Level
   1 = very tense, anxious, flushed, tremulous
   5 = overly relaxed, casual, no concern
4. Verbal Output in Test and Interview
   1 = overly taciturn, no spontaneous conversation
   5 = extremely verbose, talks when not appropriate
5. Manner of Relating to Examiner

1 = no effort to relate, withdrawn, hostile
5 = relates with too little distance, like buddy/friend
  6. Appropriateness of Behaviour
     1 = overly conforming, 'proper' behaviour
     2 = odd, unusual, or impulsive behaviour
  7. Motivation
     1 = unusually determined to be right, competitive, fearful of failure
     5 = careless, inattentive, little effort
  8. Ability to Concentrate
     1 = persists beyond need to continue, cannot shift to other activities
     5 = unable to attend to task, distracted by own ideas
  9. Confidence in Self
     1 = self-critical, seeks constant reassurance
     5 = brags of ability, satisfied with poor performance
 10. Body Type
     1 = very slender, markedly underweight
     5 = obese
 11. Rapport Established
     1 = never
     5 = at once and held throughout interview
 12. Counselling Interview Recommended
     1 = none
     2-5 = test information, counselling, interview etc.

## 4. Structured Interview Schedule (Phase II)

  1. Subject identification number
  2. Interviewer
  3. Date of interview
  4. Location of interview
  5. How old are you?
  6. Regarding present accommodations, are you living with your parents, living by yourself, or sharing accommodations?
  7. If sharing, with whom are you sharing accommodations?
  8. Where do you live?
  9. How old were you when you left the home of your parents or legal guardians to live on your own?
 10. What was the highest grade you completed in school?
 11. What program were you enrolled in?
 12. In general, how did you like school?
 13. Do you feel that you had a problem in reading, spelling, or speaking that affected your school progress?
 14. Did you have a problem with math?
 15. Do you still have that problem?

16. Has that problem affected your choice of jobs, schools, etc.?
17. Did your natural mother or father have a problem in reading, spelling, or arithmetic?
18. Did anybody else in your family have these problems?
19. Have you been attending school at all during the last five years? (if yes, code type of school, length of attendence, and whether part- or full-time)
20. What is the main purpose of school for you?
21. What were/are you studying?
22. What grade (overall) did you receive?
23. Did you complete any school degrees/diplomas/tickets in the last 5 years? (code specifics)

*Employment*

24. Are you working now?
25. If no, have you worked during the past 5 years?
26. How long did you work at your last job (or how long have you been working at your present job)?
27. What is your last/current job?
28. Is/Was it full-time?
29. Is/Was it temporary or permanent?
30. Is/Was it the kind of job you enjoy doing?
31. Is the job challenging or demanding of your talents or abilities?
32. How many jobs have you had in the last 5 years?
33. What was your approximate highest salary per month?
34. What was your salary at your longest held job?
35. Have you ever had difficulties finding a job?
36. What income do you live on?
37. Do you plan to change your job?
38. If currently unemployed, are you looking for a job that is different from that in which you worked previously?
39. What kind of job di you think you would enjoy?

*Health*

40. In the last 5 years, what health problems have you had? (code type, length, missing work or school)
41. Have you had any seizures during the last 5 years? (code type, frequency)
42. Have you had any accidents during the last 5 years?
43. Suicide attempts?
44. If yes, what kind of accident? How long were you away from school or work because of accident?
45. Do you have any health problems which prevent you from driving?

46. Have you taken any tranquilizers in the last 5 years? (code type, frequency, and duration)
47. Do you use any other prescribed medication? (code type, frequency, and duration of use)
48. Have you used any non-medical drugs during the last 5 years? If yes, what type and how often?
49. Do you drink alcoholic beverages? If yes, how often?
50. Would you describe yourself as having a problem with alcohol?
51. In the last 5 years, have you been to a speech/ hearing (eye/ear) specialist?
52. In the last 5 years, have you been to a psychologist/psychiatrist?
53. In the last 5 years, have you been to an educational/vocational counsellor?
54. Were you ever considered hyperactive? If yes, who said so?
55. Do you find yourself overly restless, or unable to settle down now?
56. Do you ever lose control of your temper?
57. Are you a fearful type of person?
58. Since we last talked to you, have you come to the attention of the police?
59. What were you charged with? What was the penalty? (code by age in sequence)

*Social Adjustment*

60. Have you ever been married or lived common-law?
61. Have you had any children? If yes to 60 and 61:
62. How many children do you have?
63. How long have you been married or lived common-law?
64. In general, how would you rate your relationship with your spouse?
65. Have you ever been separated from your spouse? (code how long after marriage, how often, divorced)
66. How would you describe your relationship with your children?
67. Do you ever physically punish your children?
68. Have you ever felt that you lost control when punishing your child?

If not married:
69. Have you ever dated? (code frequency)
70. How many close friends do you have?
71. How many casual friends do you have?
72. Are your friends equally from both sexes, more same sex, or more opposite sex?
73. Since we last talked to you, have either of your parents died?
74. Have they divorced or separated?
75. At present, how do you feel your parents get along together?
76. Is this better or worse than when you were a child?

77. Is this better or worse than when you were an adolescent or teenager?
78. How do you get along with your mother?
79. How do you get along with your father?
80. Were you physically abused as a child?
81. How do you get along with your brothers and sisters?

*Hobbies and Other than Work Activities*

82. What do you do in your spare time?
83. Are you involved with any groups or clubs? (code type and time spent there per month)
84. Do you hold any kind of office in a group or club?
85. As a child, did you enjoy athletics?
86. How competent were you?
87. Do you like reading? (how much, for pleasure or as part of job or studies)
88. Do you have a driver's licence?
89. How old were you when you first earned this?
90. Do you drive an automobile at least twice a week? (code whether for pleasure or as part of job)

*Personal Information*

91. Do you see yourself as different from other men/women of your age?
92. Do you think other people see you as being different?
93. Are you satisfied with the way your life is now?

## 5. Neurological Examination

| | HARD | SOFT |
|---|---|---|
| 1. Ataxia | Marked | Slight |
| 2. Asymmetry of skull or limbs | | |
| 3. Anosmia | Marked | Slight |
| 4. Visual Field Defect | | |
| 5. Diplopia | | |
| 6. Strabismus | | |
| 7. Saccadic Movements | | |
| 8. Nystagmus | Definite, sustained, unilateral | Unsustained, bilateral |
| 9. Dysarthria | Marked | Slight |
| 10. Dyspraxia of Tongue Movements | | |
| 11. Choreoform, Athetoid Movements | Marked | Slight |

149

| 12. | Resting Tremor | Marked | Slight |
|-----|----------------|--------|--------|
| 13. | Resting Muscle Tone | Marked spasticity or hypotonus | Mild spasticity or hypotonus uni or bilateral |
| 14. | Paresis | Asymmetrical | Slight bilateral weakness |
| 15. | Diminished or Hyperactive Tendon Reflexes | Grade 2 unilateral Grade 3 uni or bilateral | Grade 1 uni or bilateral Grade 2 bilateral exaggeration |
| 16. | Ankle Clonus | Sustained | Unsustained |
| 17. | Babinski sign | Right, left, bilateral | |
| 18. | Synkinesia | | |
| 19. | Incoordination | Marked | Slight |
| 20. | Heel/Knee testing | Marked, grade 2 uni or bilateral | Slight--grade 1 |
| 21. | Intention tremor | Marked | Slight |
| 22. | Disdiodochokinesia | Marked | Slight |
| 23. | Anaesthesia | Very Marked | Moderate or slight |
| 24. | Simultagnosia | Unilateral | Bilateral |
| 25. | Position Sense | Marked | Slight, mild |
| 26. | Graphaesthesia | | |

Do you think these findings are valid?

Yes _____ Questionable _____ No _____

Final Diagnosis        _____ Definite        Specify
of Brain               _____ Possible        Specify
Dysfunction            _____ Uncertain
                       _____ Normal

Examiner Blind  _____
Patient "gave-away"  _____

## 6. Interviewer and Test Examiner Rating Scales (Phase II)

*Scales rated by both interviewer and test examiner:*

1. Manifest anxiety level
   1-point rating: very tense, anxious, flushed, tremulous
   5-point rating: overly relaxed, casual, no concern
2. Verbal output
   1 point: overly taciturn, no spontaneous conversation
   5 points: extremely verbose, talks when not appropriate
3. Manner of relating to examiner/interviewer

150

1 point: no effort to relate, withdrawn, hostile
5 points: related with too little distance, like buddy/friend
4. Appropriateness of behaviour
   1 point: overly conforming,'proper' behaviour
   5 points: odd, unusual, or impulsive behaviour
5. Motivation
   1 point: unusually determined to be right, competitive, fearful of failure
   5 points: careless, inattentive, little effort
6. Ability to concentrate
   1 point: persists beyond need to continue, cannot shift to other activities
   5 points: unable to attend to task, distracted by own ideas
7. Confidence in self
   1 point: self-critical, seeks constant reassurance
   5 points: brags of ability, satisfied with poor performance
8. Rapport established
   1 point: never
   5 points: at once and held throughout

*Rating by Test Examiner*

9. Did participant make best effort
   1 point: tried extremely hard
   5 points: did not try at all

*Rating made jointly by interviewer and test examiner*

10. Grooming
    1 point: overly neat and orderly
    5 points: dirty, untidy, disheveled
11. Maturity of behaviour
    1 point: 'old' for age, subdued, overly serious
    5 points: childish, silly, unable to take situation seriously
12. Body type
    1 point: very slender, markedly underweight
    5 points: obese
13. Follow-up counselling by principal psychologist recommended
    1 point: none
    5 points: retest and interview necessary
14. Are the results likely to be valid?
    1 point: yes
    5 points: no

# References

Ackerman,P.T., Dykman,R.A., & Peters,J.E. (1977). Learning-disabled boys as adolescents: Cognitive factors and achievement. *Journal of the American Academy of Child Psychiatry, 16,* 296–313. (a)

Ackerman,P.T., Dykman,R.A., & Peters,J.E. (1977). Teenage status of hyperactive and nonhyperactive learning disabled boys. *American Journal of Orthopsychiatry, 47,* 577-596. (b)

Adams,R., Kocsis,J., & Estes,R.E. (1974). Soft neurological signs in learning disabled children and controls. *American Journal of Diseases of Children, 128,* 614-618.

Andrews,H., Snee, R., & Sarner, M. (1980). Graphical display of means *The American Statistician, 34,* 195-199.

Applebee,A. (1971). Research in reading retardation: Two critical problems. *Journal of Child Psychology and Psychiatry, 12,* 91-113.

Aylward,E.H. (1984). Lateral asymmetry in subgroups of dyslexic children. *Brain and Language, 22,* 221-231.

Bakker,D.J. (1979) Hemispheric differences and reading strategies: Two dyslexias? *Bulletin of the Orton Society, 29,* 84-100.

Bakker,D.J. (1984). The brain as a dependent variable. *Journal of Clinical Neuropsychology, 6,* 1-16.

Bakker,D.J. & De Wit,J. (1977). Perceptual and cortical immaturity in developmental dyslexia. In L.Tarnopol, & M.Tarnopol (Eds.), *Brain function and reading disabilities* (pp. 177-198). Baltimore: University Park Press.

Bakker,D.J., & Satz,P. (Eds.). (1970). *Specific reading disability: Advances in theory and method.* Rotterdam: Rotterdam University Press.

Balow,B., & Blomquist,M. (1965). Young adults ten to fifteen years after severe reading disability. *Elementary School Journal, 66,* 44-48.

Barlow,C.F. (1974). Soft signs in children with learning disorders. *American Journal of Diseases of Children, 128,* 605-606.

Barron,F. (1953). An ego-strength scale which predicts response to psychotherapy. *Journal of Consulting Psychology, 17,* 327-333.

Bateman,B., & Schiefelbusch,R. (1969). *Minimal brain dysfunction. (N.& SDCP Monograph, U.S. Public Health Service Publication, No.2015).* Washington, DC: U.S.Government Printing Office.

Bell,H.M. (1962). *The adjustment inventory. Revised Student Form.* Palo Alto, CA: Consulting Psychologists Press.

Benton,A.L. (1959), *Right-left discrimination and finger localization.* New York: Hoeber-Harper.

Benton,A.L., & Pearl, D. (1978). *Dyslexia: An appraisal of current knowledge.* New York: Oxford University Press.

Benton,A.L., Hamsher,K.deS., Varney,N.R. & Spreen,O. (1983). *Contributions to neuropsychological assessment.* New York: Oxford.

Berman,A. (1978). Delinquent youth and learning disabilities. In N.P.Ramos (Ed.), *Delinquent youth and learning disabilities* (pp. 48-61). San Rafael, CA: Academic Therapy.

Berman,A., & Siegal,A. (1976). A neuropsychological approach to etiology, prevention, and treatment of juvenile delinquency. In A. Davids (Ed.), *Child personality and psychopathology: Current topics. Vol. 3* (pp. 259-294). New York: Wiley.

Bingham,G. (1978). Career attitudes among boys with and without specific learning disabilities. *Exceptional Children, 44,* 341-342.

Birch,H. (Ed.). (1964). *Brain damage in children, the biological and social aspects.* Baltimore, MD: Williams and Wilkins.

Black, F.W.(1974) Patterns of cognitive impairment in children with suspected and documented neurological dysfunction. *Perceptual and Motor Skills, 39,* 115-120.

Blalock,J.W. (1982). Residual learning disabilities in young adults: Implications for rehabilitation. *Journal of Applied Rehabilitation Counselling, 13,* 9-13.

Blashfield,R.K. (1980). Propositions regarding the use of cluster analysis in clinical research. *Journal of Consulting and Clinical Psychology, 48,* 456-459.

Blishen,B.J., & McRoberts,H. (1976). A revised socioeconomic index for occupations in Canada. *Canadian Review of Sociology and Anthropology, 13,* 71-79.

Boder,E. (1970). Developmental dyslexia: A new diagnostic approach based on the identification of three subtypes. *Journal of School Health, 40,* 289-290.

Boll,T.J., & Reitan,R.M. (1972). Motor and tactile-perceptual deficits in brain-damaged children. *Perceptual and Motor Skills, 34,* 343-350.

Borland,B.L., & Heckman,H.K. (1976). Hyperactive boys and their brothers. *Archives of General Psychiatry, 33,* 669-675.

Bray,G. (1976). *The obese patient, Vol. IX.* Philadelphia: W.B. Saunders Co.

Brim,O.G., & Kagan,J. (Eds.). (1980). *Constancy and change in human development.* Cambridge: Harvard University Press.

Broman,S.H., Nichols,P.L., & Kennedy,W. (1975). *Pre-school IQ: Prenatal and early developmental correlates.* Hillsdale, NJ: Lawrence Erlbaum.

Bruck,M. (1985). The adult functioning of children with specific learning disabilities: A follow-up study. In I.E.Sigel (Ed.), *Advances in applied developmental psychology, Vol.1,* pp. 91-129. Norwood, NJ: Ablex.

Bryan,T. & Bryan,J. (1975). *Understanding learning disabilities.* New York: Alfred Publishing Company.

Bryan,T. (1974). Peer popularity of learning disabled children. *Journal of Learning Disabilities, 7,* 261-268.

Burnside,B. (1986). *Learning disabled children growing up: Emotional adjustment in adulthood. Unpublished doctoral dissertation,* University of Victoria.

Cattell,R.B. (1978). *The scientific use of factor analysis in the behavioral and life sciences.* New York: Plenum Press.

CELDIC (The Commission on Emotional and Learning Disorders in Children). (1970). *One million children: A national study of Canadian children with emotional and learning disorders. L. Crainford.*

Chall,J.S., & Mirsky,A.F. (Eds.). (1978). *Education and the brain. (The 77th Yearbook of the National Society for the Study of Education Part II).* Chicago: University of Chicago Press.

Chapman,J.W., & Boersma,F.J. (1980). *Affective correlates of learning disabilities.* Lisse, Netherlands: Swets & Zeitlinger.

Childs,B., Finucci,J.M., Pulver,A.E., & Tielsch,J.(1982). *The natural history of specific reading disability; education outcomes.* Unpublished manuscript, Baltimore, MD: Department of Pediatrics, Johns Hopkins University.

Christiansen,K.O. (1977). A review of studies of criminality mong twins. In S.A. Mednick, & K.O. Christiansen (Eds.), *Biosocial bases of criminal behavior* (pp. 45-88). New York: Gardner Press.

Clark,C.M., & Spreen, O. (1983). Psychometric properties of dichotic words tests. *Journal of Clinical Neuropsychology, 5,* 169-179.

154

Clements,S.D. (1966). Minimal brain dysfunction in children -Terminology and identification. *NINDB Monograph No. 3. Washington, DC: U.S. Department of Health, Education, and Welfare.*

Clements,S.D., & Peters,J.E. (1963). Minimal brain dysfunction in the school-age child. *Archives of General Psychiatry, 6,* 185-197.

Colligan,R.C., Osborne,D., Swenson,W.M., & Offord,K.P. (1983). *The MMPI: A contemporary normative study.* New York: Praeger.

Compton,R.E. (1974). Diagnostic evaluation of committed delinquents. In B.L.Kratoville (Ed.), *Youth in trouble* (pp. 68-75). San Rafael, CA: Academic Therapy.

Connolly,C. (1969). The psychosocial adjustment of children with dyslexia. *Exceptional Children, 36,* 126-127.

Conry,R., & Plant,W.T. (1965). WAIS and group test predictions of an academic success criterion. High school and college. *Educational and Psychological Measurement, 25,* 493-500.

Cordoni,B.K., O'Donnell,J.P., Ramaniah,N.V., Kurtz,J., & Rosensheim,K. (1981). Wechsler adult intelligence score patterns for learning disabled young adults. *Journal of Learning Disabilities, 14,* 404-407.

Cruickshank,W.M. (Ed.). (1966). *The teacher of brain-injured children.* Syracuse, NY: Syracuse University Press.

Cruickshank,W.M. (1971). *Psychology of exceptional children and youth.* Englewood Cliffs, NJ: Prentice-Hall.

Cruickshank,W.M. (1979). Learning disabilities: A definitional statement. In E. Polak, (Ed.), *Issues and Initiatives in learning disabilities: Selected papers from the First National Conference on Learning Disabilities* (pp. 15-42). Ottawa: Canadian Association for Children with Learning Disabilities.

Culver,C.M. (1969) Test of right-left discrimination. *Perceptual and Motor Skills, 29,* 863-867.

de la Cruz,F.F., Fox,B.H., & Roberts,R.H. (Eds.). (1973). Minimal brain dysfunction. *Annals of the New York Academy of Sciences, 205.*

Decker,S.N. (1982). Reading disability: Is there a hereditary pattern? In R.N.Malatesha & L.C.Hartlage (Eds.), *Neuropsychology and cognition, Vol.2.* The Hague: Martinus Nijhoff.

Decker,S.N. & DeFries, J.C. (1981). Cognitive ability profiles in families of reading-disabled children. *Developmental Medicine and Child Neurology, 23,* 217-227.

Denbigh,K. (1979). *Neurological impairment and educational achievement: A follow-up of learning disabled children. Unpublished M.A. Thesis,* University of Victoria.

Denckla,M.B. (1977). Minimal brain dysfunction and dyslexia: Beyond diagnosis by exclusion. In M.E. Blaw, I. Rapin, & M. Kinsbourne (Eds.), *Topics in child neurology* (pp. 243-262). New York: Spectrum Publications.

Denhoff,E. (1973). The natural life history of children with minimal brain dysfunction. *Annals of the New York Academy of Sciences, 205,* 188-205.

Deutsch,C.P., & Schumer,F. (1970). *Brain-damaged children: A Modality-oriented exploration of performance.* New York, NY: Brunner/Mazel.

Diaconis,P., & Efron,B. (1983). Computer-intensive methods in statistics. *Scientific American, 248,* 116-130.

Doehring,D.G. (1968). *Patterns of impairment in specific reading disabilities.* Bloomington, IN: Indiana University Press.

Doehring,D.G., & Hoshko,I.M. (1977). Classification of reading problems by the Q technique of factor analysis. *Cortex, 13,* 281-294.

Doehring,D.G., Trites, R.L., Patel, P.G., & Fiedorowicz, A.M. (1981). *Reading disabilities: The interaction of reading, language, and neuropsychological deficits.* New York: Academic Press.

Duling,F., Eddy,S., & Risko,V. (1970). *Learning disabilities of juvenile delinquents.* Morgantown, WV: Department of Educational Services, R.F. Kennedy Youth Center.

155

Dunn,L.M., & Markwardt, F.C., Jr. (1970). *Manual: Peabody Individual Achievement Test.* Circle Pines, MN: American Guidance Service.

Dykman,R.A., Peters, J.E., & Ackerman, P.T. (1973). Experimental approaches to the study of minimal brain dysfunction: A follow-up study. *Annals of the New York Academy of Sciences 205,* 93-107.

Eling,P. (1983). Comparing different measures of laterality: Do they relate to a single mechanism? *Journal of Clinical Neuropsychology, 5,* 135-147.

Elliott,D.S. (1984). A longitudinal study of delinquency and dropouts. In S.A.Mednick, M.Harway, & K.M.Finello (Eds.), *Handbook of longitudinal research, Vol.2* (pp. 422-438). New York: Praeger.

Ensminger,M.E., Kellam,S.G., & Rubin,B.R. (1983). School and family origins of delinquency: comparison by sex. In K.T.Van Dusen & S.A.Mednick (Eds.), *Prospective studies of crime and deliquency* (pp. 73-97). Boston: Kluwer-Nijhoff.

Farrington,D.P. (1983). Offending from 10 to 25 years of age. In K.T.Van Dusen & S.A.Mednick (Eds.), *Prospective studies of crime and delinquency* (pp. 17-37). Boston: Kluwer-Nijhoff.

Filskov,S.B., & Leli,D.A. (1981). Assessment of the individual in neuropsychological practice. In S.B. Filskov & T.J. Boll (Eds.), *Handbook of clinical neuropsychology* (pp. 545-576). New York: Wiley.

Finucci,J. & Childs,B. (1981). Are there really more dyslexic boys than girls? In A. Ansara, N. Geshwind, A. Galaburda, M. Albert, & N. Gartrell (Eds.), *Sex differences in dyslexia* (pp. 1-10). Baltimore, MD: Orton Dyslexia Society.

Fisk,J.L., & Rourke,B.P. (1979). Identification of subtypes of learning disabled children at three age levels: A neuropsychological, multivariate approach. *Journal of Clinical Neuropsychology, 1,* 289-310.

Fisk,J.L., & Rourke,B.P. (1984 February). *Personality subtypes of learning disabled children: Two validation studies.* Paper presented at the Meeting of the International Neuropsychological Society, Houston, Tx.

Flor-Henry,P. (1976). Lateralized temporal-limbic dysfunction and psychopathology. *Annals of the New York Academy of Sciences, 280,* 777-795.

Gaddes,W.H. (1976). Prevalence estimates and the need for definition of learning disabilities. In R.M. Knights & D.L. Bakker (Eds.), *The neuropsychology of learning disorders, theoretical approaches* (pp. 3-24). Baltimore, MD: University Park Press.

Gaddes,W.H. (1984). *Learning disabilities and brain function, a neuropsychological approach (2nd ed.).* New York: Springer.

Gaddes,W.H., & Crockett, D. (1975). The Spreen-Benton aphasia tests: Normative data as a measure of normal language development. *Brain and Language, 5,* 257-280.

Gesell,A., & Armatruda,C. (1947). *Developmental diagnosis.* New York: Hoeber.

Gottesman,R. (1979). Follow up of learning disabled children. *Learning Disability Quarterly, 2,* 60-69.

Gottesman,R., Belmont,I., & Kaminer,R. (1975). Admission and follow-up status of reading disabled children referred to a medical clinic. *Journal of Learning Disabilities, 8,* 642-650.

Gottfredson,L., Finucci,J. & Childs,B. (1983). *Adult occupational success of dyslexic boys: Long-term followup.* (Center for study of social organizations of schools. Report No.334). March 1983.

Graham,F.K., Ernhart,C.B., Thurston,D., & Craft,M. (1962). Development three years after perinatal anoxia and other potentially damaging newborn experiences. *Psychological Monographs, 76,* 522.

Graham,F.K., Ernhart,C.B., Craft,M., & Berman,P.W. (1963). Brain injury in the preschool child: Some developmental considerations-I. Performance of normal children. *Psychological Monographs, 77,* 573.

Greenberg,L., & McMahon,S. (1977). Serial neurological examination of hyperactive children. *Pediatrics, 59,* 584-587.

156

Halstead,W.C. (1947). *Brain and intelligence.* Chicago: University of Chicago Press.

Hanvik,L.J., Nelson,S.E., Hanson,H.B., Anderson,A.S., Dressler, W.H., & Zarling,V.R. (1961). Diagnosis of cerebral dysfunction in child; as made in a child guidance clinic. *American Journal of Diseases of Children, 101,* 364-375.

Harris,R.E., & Lingoes,J.C. (1968). *Subscales for the MMPI: An aid to profile interpretation.* University of California, San Francisco, Department of Psychiatry, 1955 (Mimeo); corrected version.

Harway,M. Mednick,S.A., & Mednick,B. (1984). Research strategies: Methodological and practical problems. In S.A.Mednick, M.Harway, & K.M.Finello (Eds.), *Handbook of longitudinal research, Vol.1* (pp. 22-30). New York: Praeger.

Hechtman,L., Weiss,G., Finklestein,J., Werner,A., & Benn,R. (1976). Hyperactives as young adults: Preliminary report. *Canadian Medical Association Journal, 115,* 625-630.

Helper,M.M. (1980). Follow-up of children with minimal brain dysfunctions; outcomes and predictors. In H.E. Rie, & E.D. Rie (Eds.), *Handbook of minimal brain dysfunctions, a critical review* (pp. 75-114). New York: Wiley.

Herbst,A., & Roesler,H.D. (1986). *Frühkindlich Hirngeschädigte als Erwachsene (Early infant brain damaged subjects as adults).* Leipzig: Hirzel.

Herjanic,B.M., & Penick,E.C. (1972). Adult outcome of disabled child readers. *Journal of Special Education, 6,* 397-410.

Hern,A. (1979). *Health and behavioral adjustment in later life for learning handicapped children with and without neurological impairment.* M.A. thesis, University of Victoria.

Hern,A. (1984). *Neurological signs in learning disabled children: Persistence over time, and incidence in adulthood compared to normal learners.* Doctoral dissertation, University of Victoria.

Hern,A., & Spreen,O. (1984 February). *Persistence and incidence of neurological findings in learning disabled and normal learning subjects from age 10 to early adulthood.* Paper presented at the meeting of the International Neuropsychological Society, Houston, TX.

Hern,A., & Spreen,O. (in press). Health adjustment in learning handicapped children: A follow-up study. *Developmental Medicine and Child Neurology.*

Hertzig,M.E., & Birch,H.G. (1968). Neurological organization in psychiatrically disturbed adolescents: A comparative consideration of sex differences. *Archives of General Psychiatry, 19,* 528-538.

Hertzig,M.E., Bortner,M., & Birch,H.G. (1969). Neurological findings in children educationally designated as brain damaged. *American Journal of Orthopsychiatry, 39,* 437-446.

Howden,M.E. (1967). *A nineteen-year follow-up study of good, average and poor readers in the fifth and sixth grades.* Doctoral dissertation, Eugene: University of Oregon.

Isaacson,R.L. (1968). *The neuropsychology of development.* New York: John Wiley.

Jastak,J., & Jastak,R. (1978). *Manual: The Wide Range Achievement Test.* Wilmington, DE: Jastak Associates.

Jessor,R., & Jessor,S.L. (1984). Adolescence to young adulthood: A twelve-year prospective study of problem behavior and psychosocial development. In S.A.Mednick, M.Harway & K.M. Finello (Eds.), *Handbook of longitudinal research, Vol.2.* (pp. 34-61). New York: Praeger.

Johnson,D., & Myklebust,H. (1967). *Learning disabilities: Educational principles and practices.* New York: Grune and Stratton.

Johnson,E.L., & Neumann,C. (1975). Multidisciplinary evaluation of learning behavior problems in children. *Journal of Ostheopathic Association, 74,* 168-174.

Kaspar,J.C., Millichap,J.G., Backus,R., Child,D., & Schulman,J.L. (1971). Study of the relationship between neurological evidence of brain damage in children and activity and distractibility. *Journal of Consulting and Clinical Psychology, 36,* 329-337.

Kaste,C.M. (1972). A ten-year followup of children diagnosed in a child guidance clinic as having cerebral dysfunction. *Dissertation Abstracts International, 33,* 1797-1798.

Katz-Garris,L., McCue,M., Garris,R.P., & Herring,J. (1983). Psychiatric rehabilitation: An outcome study. *Rehabilitation Counselling Bulletin, 26,* 329-335.

157

Kinsbourne,M. (1973). Minimal brain dysfunction as a neurodevelopmental lag. *Annals of the New York Academy of Sciences, 205,* 268-273.

Kirkegaard-Sorensen,L., & Mednick,S.A.(1977). A prospective study of predictors of criminality: 4.School behavior. In S.A. Mednick & K.O. Christiansen (Eds.), *Biosocial bases of criminal behavior* (pp. 255-266). New York: Gardner Press.

Kleinpeter,U., & Goellnitz,G. (1976). Achievement and adaptation disorders in brain-damaged children. *International Journal of Mental Health, 4,* 19-35.

Klonoff,A., & Low,M. (1974). Disordered brain function in young children and early adolescents; neuropsychological and electroencephalographic correlates. In R.M. Reitan, & L.A. Davison, (Eds.), *Clinical neuropsychology: Current status and applications* (pp. 121-178). Washington: V.H.Winston.

Koppitz,E.M. (1971). *Children with learning disabilities: A five year follow-up study.* New York: Grune and Stratton.

Krynicki,V.E. (1978). Cerebral dysfunction in repetitively assaultive adolescents. *Journal of Nervous and Mental Diseases, 166,* 59-67.

LaBreche,T.M. (1982). *The Victoria revision of the Halstead Category Test. Unpublished doctoral dissertation,* University of Victoria.

Lai,C. (1982). *Hierarchical grouping analysis with optional contiguity constraint. Program Manual, Computing Services,* University of British Columbia.

Larrabee,G.J., Kane,R.L., & Schuck,J.R. (1983). Factor analysis of the WAIS and Wechsler Memory Scale: An analysis of the construct validity of the Wechler Memory Scale. *Journal of Clinical Neuropsychology, 5,* 159-168.

Laufer,M.W. (1971). Long-term management and some follow-up findings on the use of drugs with minimal cerebral syndrome. *Journal of Learning Disabilities, 4,* 518-522.

Levine,M.D., Brooks,R., & Shonkoff,J. (1980). *A pediatric approach to learning disorders.* New York: Wiley.

Lewis, D.O., & Balla, D.A. (1976). *Delinquency and psychopathology.* New York: Grune and Stratton.

Loney,J., Kramer,J., & Milich,R. (1984). The hyperkinetic child grows up: Predictors of symptoms, delinquency, and achievement at follow-up. In S.A.Mednick, M.Harway, & K.M.Finello (Eds.), *Handbook of longitudinal research, Vol.1* (pp. 426-447). New York: Praeger.

Loney,J., Whaley-Klahn,M.A., Kosier,T., & Conboy,J. (1983). Hyperactive boys and their brothers at 21: Predictors of aggressive and antisocial outcomes. In K.T.Van Dusen & S.A.Mednick (Eds.), *Prospective studies of crime and delinquency* (pp. 181-207). Boston: Kluwer-Nijhoff.

Lorr,M. (1983). *Cluster analysis for social scientists.* San Francisco: Jossey-Bass.

Lovett,M W. (1984). A developmental perspective on reading dysfunction: Accuracy and rate criteria in the subtyping of dyslexic children. *Brain and Language, 22,* 67-91.

Lunneborg,C.E. (1985). Estimating the correlation coefficient: The bootstrap approach. *Psychological Bulletin, 98,* 209-215.

Lyon,R., & Watson,B. (1981). Empirically derived subgroups of learning disabled readers: Diagnostic characteristics. *Journal of Learning Disabilities, 14,* 256-261.

MacAndrew,C. (1965). The differentiation of male alcoholic outpatients from nonalcohol psychiatric outpatients by means of the MMPI. *Quarterly Journal of Studies of Alcohol, 26,* 238-246.

Marshall,J.C., & Newcombe,F. (1973). Patterns of paralexia: A psycholinguistic approach. *Developmental Medicine and Child Neurology, 2,* 175-199.

Marshall,J.C., Caplan,D. and Holmes,J.M. (1975). The measure of laterality. *Neuropsychologia, 13,* 315-321.

Matarazzo,J.D. (1972). *Wechsler's measurement and appraisal of adult intelligence (5th and enlarged edition).* Baltimore: Williams & Wilkins.

Matarazzo,J.D., & Herman,D.O. (1984). Base rate data for the WAIS-R: Test-retest stability and VIQ-PIQ differences. *Journal of Clinical Neuropsychology, 6,* 351-366.

158

Mattis,S., French,J., & Rapin,I. (1975).Dyslexia in children and young adults: Three independent neuropsychological syndromes. *Developmental Medicine and Child Neurology, 17,* 150-163.

Mauser,A.J. (1974). Learning disabilities and delinquent youth. *Academic Therapy, 9,* 389-402.

Maxwell,A.E. (1971). Multivariate statistical methods and classification problems. *British Journal of Psychiatry, 119,* 121-127.

McAllister,M., & Spreen,O. (1981). *Victoria norms for grades one to five on the WISC, WRAT and PPVT. Unpublished manuscript,* University of Victoria.

McDermott,P.A. (1981). The manifestations of problem behaviour in ten age groups of Canadian school children. *Canadian Journal of Behavioural Science, 13,* 310-319.

Mednick,B.R. (1973). Breakdown in high-risk subjects: Familial and early environmental factors. *Journal of Abnormal Psychology, 82,* 469-475.

Mendelson,W., Johnson,N., & Stewart,M. (1971). Hyperactive children as teenagers: A follow-up study. *Journal of Nervous and Mental Diseases, 153,* 272-279.

Menkes,M.M., Rowe,J.S., & Menkes,J.H. (1967). A twenty-five year follow-up study on the hyperkinetic child with minimal brain dysfunction. *Pediatrics, 39,* 393-399.

Minde,K., Lewin,D., Weiss,G., Lavigueur,H., Douglas,V., & Sykes,E. (1971). The hyperactive child in elementary school: A five-year, controlled follow-up. *Exceptional Children, 38,* 215-221.

Minde,K.G., Weiss,G., & Mendelson,N. (1972). A five-year follow-up study on the hyperkinetic child with minimal brain dysfunction. *Journal of the American Academy of Child Psychiatry, 11,* 595-610.

Minskoff,J.G. (1973). Differential approaches to prevalence estimates of learning disabilities. *Annals of the New York Academy of Sciences, 205,* 139-145.

Mojena,R., & Wishart,D. (1980). Stopping rules for Ward's clustering method. Compsat: 1980. *Proceedings in Computational Statistics. Fourth Symposium.* Vienna: Physica-Verlag.

Morris,R., Blashfield,R., & Satz,P. (1981). Neuropsychology and cluster analysis: Potentials and problems. *Journal of Clinical Neuropsychology, 3,* 79-99.

Muehl,S., & Forell,E.R. (1973-1974). A followup study of disabled readers: Variables related to high school reading performance. *Reading Research Quarterly, 9,* 110-123.

Myklebust,H. (1973). Identification and diagnosis of children with learning disabilities: An interdisciplinary study of criteria. In S. Walzer, & P. Wolff (Eds.), *Minimal cerebral dysfunction in children* (pp. 55-77). New York: Grune & Stratton.

Myklebust,H.R., Boshes,B., Olson,D.A., & Cole,C.H. (1969). *Minimal brain damage in children (Final report).* Washington, DC: Department of Health, Education, and Welfare.

National Advisory Committee on Handicapped Children. (1968). *Special education for handicapped children (First Annual Report).* Washington, DC: U.S. Department of Health, Education, and Welfare, Office of Education.

Nesselroade,J.R., & Delhees,K.H. (1966). Methods and findings in experimentally based personality theory. In R.B.Cattell (Ed.), *Handbook of multivariate experimental psychology* (pp. 563-610). Chicago: Rand McNally.

Nesselroade,J.R., Stigler,S.M., & Baltes,P.B. (1980). Regression toward the mean and the study of change. *Psychological Bulletin, 88,* 622-637.

Nichols,P.L., & Chen,T.C. (1981). *Minimal brain dysfunction, a prospective study.* Hillsdale, NJ: Lawrence Earlbaum Associates.

Nissen,G. (1980). Medizinische Aspekte der Lernbehinderung (Medical aspects of learning disability). In G.O.Kanter & O.Speck (Eds.), *Handbuch der Sonderpaedagogik/Paedagogik der Lernbehinderten.* Berlin: Marhold.

Obrzut,J.E., Obrzut,A., Bryden,M.P., & Bartels,S.G. (1985). Information processing and speech lateralization in learning-disabled children. *Brain and Language, 25,* 87-101.

O'Connor,S.C., & Spreen,O. (1987). The relationship between parent's socioeconomic status and education level with learning disabled children's long-term occupational and educational achievement. *Journal of Clinical and Experimental Neuropsychology, 9,* 27.

159

Offord,D., Marohn,R.C., & Ostrov,E. (1983). *The psychological world of the juvenile delinquent.* New York: Academic Press.

Offord,D.R., Poushinsky,M.F., & Sullivan,K. (1978). School performance, IQ and delinquency. *British Journal of Criminology, 18,* 110-127.

Ondarza-Landwehr,G. von (1979). *Prognose minimaler Hirnfunktionsstörungen im Vorschulalter (Prognosis of minimal brain dysfunction).* Weinheim, Germany: Beltz.

Orton,S.T.(1937). *Reading, writing and speech problems in children.* New York: Norton.

Ozols,E.J., & Rourke,B.P.(1985). Dimensions of social sensi-tivity in two types of learning disabled children. In B.P.Rourke (Ed.), *Neuropsychology of learning disabilities: Essentials of subtype analysis* (pp. 281-307). New York: Guilford.

Page-El,E., & Grossman,H.J. (1973). Neurologic appraisal in learning disorders. *Pediatric Clinics of North America, 20,* 599-605.

Page,S., & Steffi,R. (1984). WAIS and WISC-R 'VP' scores: Sampling characteristics from three psychiatric populations. *Canadian Journal of Behavioural Science, 16,* 99-106.

Pasamanick,B., & Knobloch,H. (1960). Brain damage and reproductive asualty. *American Journal of Orthopsychiatry, 30,* 298-305.

Peter,B.M., & Spreen,O. (1979). Behavior rating and personal adjustment scales of neurologically and learning handicapped children during adolescence and early adulthood: Results of a follow-up study. *Journal of Clinical Neuropsychology 1,* 75-92.

Peters,J.E., Romine,J.S., & Dykman,R.A. (1975). A special neurological examination of children with learning disabilities. *Developmental Medicine and Child Neurology, 17,* 63-78.

Phillips,J.C., & Kelley,D.H. (1979). School failure and delinquency: Which causes which? *Criminology, 17,* 194-207.

Pincus,J.H., Lewis,D.O., Shanok,S.S., & Glaser,G.H. (1979). Neurologic abnormalities in violent delinquents. *Neurology, 29,* 586.

Pirozzolo,F.J. (1979). *The neuropsychology of developmental reading disorders.* New York: Praeger.

Polloway,E.A., Smith,J.D., & Patton,J.R. (1984). Learning disabilities: An adult developmental perspective. *Learning Disability Quarterly, 7,* 179-186.

Porter,J.E., & Rourke,B.P. (1985). Socio-emotional functioning of learning disabled children: A subtypal analysis of personality patterns. In B.P. Rourke (Ed.), *Neuropsychology of learning disabilities: Essentials of subtype analysis.* (pp. 257-279). New York: Guilford.

Preston,R., & Yarington,D.J. (1967). Status of fifty retarded readers eight years after reading clinic diagnosis. *Journal of Reading, 11,* 122-129.

Purdue Research Foundation. (1948). Examiner's manual for the Purdue Pegboard. Chicago: Science Research Associates.

Rawson,M. (1968). *Developmental language disability: Adult accomplishment of dyslexic boys.* Baltimore: Johns Hopkins University Press.

Robinson,H.M., & Smith,H.K. (1972). Reading clinic clients - Ten years after. *Elementary School Journal, 63,* 22-27.

Rollett,B., & Bartram,M. (Eds.). (1976). *Einfuehrung in die hierarchische Clusteranalyse (Introduction to hierarchical cluster analysis).* Stuttgart: Klett.

Rourke,B.P. (Ed.). (1985). *Neuropsychology of learning disabilities: Essentials of subtype analysis.* New York: Guilford.

Rourke,B.P., & Fisk,J.L. (1981). Socio-emotional disturbances of learning disabled children: The role of central processing deficits. *Bulletin of the Orton Society, 31,* 77-88.

Rourke,B.P., & Orr,R.R. (1977). Prediction of the reading and spelling performances of normal and retarded readers: A 4 year follow up. *Journal of Abnormal Child Psychology, 5,* 9-20.

Rourke,B.P., & Strang,J.D. (1983). Subtypes of reading and arithmetical disabilities: A neuropsychological analysis. In M. Rutter (Ed.), *Developmental neuropsychiatry* (pp. 473-488). New York: Guilford Press.

Rubin,R., & Balow,B. (1971). Learning and behavior disorders: A longitudinal study. *Exceptional children, 38,* 293-299.

Russell,V. (1984). *The emotional adjustment of a learning disabled population in adulthood, as measured by the Minnesota Multiphasic Personality Inventory. M.A.Thesis:* University of Victoria.

Russell,V., & Spreen,O. (1984 February). *The emotional adjustment of a learning disabled population in adulthood as measured by the MMPI.* Paper presented at the meeting of the International Neuropsychological Society, Houston, TX.

Rutter,M. (1978). Prevalence and types of dyslexia. In A.L. Benton & D. Pearl (Eds.), *Dyslexia: An appraisal of current knowledge* (pp. 4-28). New York: Oxford University Press.

Rutter,M. (1982). Syndromes attributed to minimal brain dysfunction in childhood. *American Journal of Psychiatry, 139,* 21-33.

Rutter,M., & Giller,H. (1983). *Juvenile delinquency: Trends and perspectives.* New York: Guilford.

Rutter,M , Graham,P,, & Yule,W. (1970). *A neuropsychiatric study in childhood. (Clinics in Developmental Medicine No.35-36).* Philadelphia: J.B.Lippincott. (a)

Rutter,M., Tizard,J., & Whitmore,K. (Eds.). (1970). *Education, health, and behavior.* London: Longmans. (b)

Salter,K. (1983). *Handedness in a clinic-referred sample of disabled learners as a function of neurological involvement. Unpublished M.A.Thesis,* University of Victoria.

Salter,K., & Spreen,O. (1984). *Handedness in a clinic referred sample of disabled learners as a function of neurological involvement.* Paper presented at the International Neuropsychological Society Meeting, Houston, TX.

Sarazin,F., & Spreen,O. (1986). Fifteen year reliability of some neuropsychological tests in learning disabled subjects with and without neurological impairment. *Journal of Clinical and Experimental Neuropsychology, 8,* 190-200.

Sarle,W.S. (1982). Documentation for SAS clustering routine. In *SAS user's guide: Statistics,* Cary, North Carolina: SAS Institute.

Satz,P., & Fletcher,J.M. (1980). Minimal brain dysfunction: An appraisal of research concepts and methods. In H.E. Rie & E.D. Rie (Eds.), *Handbook of minimal brain dysfunction* (pp. 669-714). New York: Wiley.

Satz,P., & Morris,R. (1981). Learning disability subtypes: A review. In F.J. Pirozzolo & M.C. Wittrock (Eds.), *Neuropsychological and cognitive processes in reading* (pp. 109-141). New York: Academic Press.

Satz,P., Taylor,H.G., Friel,J., & Fletcher,J.M. (1978). Some developmental and predictive precursors of reading disabilities: A six-year followup. In A.Benton & D.Pearl (Eds.), *Dyslexia: A critical appraisal of current theory* (pp. 313-348). New York: Oxford University Press.

Schmitt,B.C. (1975). The minimal brain dysfunction myth. *American Journal of Diseases of Children, 129,* 1313-1318.

Schonhaut,S., & Satz,P. (1983). Prognosis for children with learning disabilities. A review of the follow-up studies. In M. Rutter (Ed.), *Developmental Neuropsychiatry.* (pp. 542-563). New York: Guilford Press.

Schulsinger,H. (1976). A ten-year follow-up of schizophrenic mothers. *Acta Psychiatrica Scandinavica, 53,* 371-386.

Shankweiler,D. (1964). Developmental dyslexia: A critique and review of recent evidence. *Cortex, 1,* 53-62.

Silver,A.A., & Hagin,R.A. (1963). Specific reading disability: A twelve year follow-up study. *American Journal of Orthopsychiatry, 33,* 338-339.

Silver,A.A., & Hagin,R.A. (1964). Specific reading disability: Follow-up studies. *American Journal of Orthopsychiatry, 34,* 95-102.

Silverman,L.J., & Metz,A.S. (1973). Number of pupils with specific learning disabilities in local public schools in the United States: Spring 1970. *Annals of the New York Academy of Sciences, 205,* 146-157.

Spreen,O. (1978). *Learning disabled children growing up (Final Report).* Canada Health and Welfare. University of Victoria, Monograph. (a).

161

Spreen,O. (1981). The relationship between learning disability, neurological impairment and delinquency: Results of a follow-up. *Journal of Nervous and Mental Diseases, 169,* 791-799.

Spreen,O. (1982). Adult outcomes of reading disorders. In R.N. Malatesha & P.G. Aaron (Eds.), *Reading disorders: Varieties and treatments* (pp. 473-498). New York: Academic Press.

Spreen,O. (1983). *Learning disabled children growing up: A follow-up into adulthood.* University of Victoria Monograph. (a)

Spreen,O. (1983). Learning disabled children growing up. In G.Schwartz (Ed.), *Advances in research & services for children with special needs* (pp. 69-75). Vancouver: University of British Columbia Press. (b).

Spreen,O. (1984). A prognostic view from middle childhood. In M. Levine & P. Satz (Eds.), *Middle childhood: Developmental variations and dysfunction* (pp. 405-432). New York: Academic Press.

Spreen,O. (1986). Attention deficit syndrome in learning-disabled children: Relation with neurological findings and outcome in young adulthood. *Journal of Clinical and Experimental Neuropsychology, 8,* 121-122.

Spreen,O., & Benton,A.L. (1967,1977). *The Neurosensory Center Comprehensive Examination for Aphasia.* University of Victoria.

Spreen,O., & Gaddes,W.H. (1969). Developmental norms for 15 neuropsychological tests age 6 to 15. *Cortex, 5,* 171-191.

Spreen,O., & Haaf,R.G. (1986). Empirically derived learning disability subtypes: A replication attempt and longitudinal patterns over 15 years. *Journal of Learning Disabilities, 19,* 170-180.

Spreen,O., & Lawriw,I. (1980). *Neuropsychological tests results as predictors of outcome of learning handicap in late adolescence and early adult years.* Paper, International Neuropsychological Society Meeting, San Francisco, CA.

Starfield,B. & Pless,I.B.(1980). Physical health. In O.G. Brim, & J. Kagan (Eds.), *Constancy and change in human development* (pp. 272-324). Cambridge: Harvard University Press.

Statistics Canada, *Canada Employment & Immigration. Victoria, B.C. (personal communication).*

Stein,D.G., & Dawson,R.G. (1980). The dynamics of growth, organization and adaptability in the central nervous system. In O.G. Brim, & J. Kagan (Eds.), *Constancy and Change in Human Development* (pp. 163-228). Cambridge: Harvard University Press.

Stein,K.B. (1968). The TSC scales: The outcome of a cluster analysis of 550 MMPI items. In P. McReynolds (Ed.), *Advances in psychological assessment (Vol. 1).* Palo Alto, CA: Science and Behavior Books.

Strang,J.D. (1981). *Factors influencing the personality adjustment of learning disabled children. Ph.D. dissertation:* University of Windsor.

Strauss,A.A., & Kephart,N.C. (1955). *Psychopathology and education of the brain-injured child. Vol.II: Progress in theory and clinic.* New York: Grune & Stratton.

Strauss,A.A., & Lethinen,L. (1947). *Psychopathology and education of the brain-injured child.* New York: Grune & Stratton.

Tarnopol,L., & Tarnopol,M. (Eds.). (1977). *Brain function and reading disabilities.* Baltimore: University Park Press.

Taylor,J.A. (1953). A personality scale of manifest anxiety. *Journal of Abnormal and Social Psychology, 48,* 285-290.

Thurstone,R. (1938). *Primary mental abilities.Chicago:* University of Chicago Press.

Trites,R., & Fiedorowicz,C. (1976). Follow-up study of children with specific (or primary) reading disability. In R.Knights & D.J. Bakker (Eds.), *The neuropsychology of learning disorders: Theoretical approaches* (pp. 41-50). Baltimore, MD: University Park Press.

Tucker,D. (1981). Lateral brain function, emotion, and conceptualization. *Psychological Bulletin, 89,* 19-46.

Tuokko,H.A. (1982). *Cognitive correlates of arithmetic performance in clinic referred children. Unpublished doctoral dissertation,* University of Victoria.

Vierkunen,M., & Nuutila,A. (1976). Specific reading retardation, hyperactive child syndrome, and juvenile delinquency. *Acta Psychiatrica Scandinavica, 54,* 25-28.

Vierkunen,M., Nuutila,A., & Huusko,S. (1976). Effect of brain injury on social adaptability; longitudinal study on frequency of criminality. *Acta Psychiatrica Scandinavica, 53,* 168-172.

Ward,J. (1963). Hierarchical grouping to optimize an objective function. *Journal of the American Statistical Association, 58,* 236-244.

Washburn,W.Y. (1975). Where to go in Voc-Ed for secondary LD students. *Academic Therapy, 11,* 31-35.

Watson,B.U., Goldgar, D.E., & Ryschon, K.L. (1983). Subtypes of reading disability. *Journal of Clinical Neuropsychology, 5,* 377-399.

Wechsler,D. (1974). *Manual for the WISC-R.* New York: The Psychological Corporation.

Wechsler,D. (1981). *Manual for the WAIS-R.* New York: The Psychological Corporation.

Wechsler,D., & Stone,C.P. (1945). *Manual: The Wechsler Memory Scale.* New York: The Psychological Corporation.

Weiss,G., Minde,K., Werry,J.S., Douglas,V., & Nemeth,E. (1971). Studies on the hyperactive child-VIII: Five-year follow-up. *Archives of General Psychiatry, 24,* 409-414.

Wender,P.H. (1971). *Minimal brain dysfunction in children.* New York: Wiley.

Werner,E.E., & Smith,R.S. (1977). *Kauai's children come of age.* Honolulu: University Press of Hawaii.

Werry,J.S., Minde,K., Guzman,A., Weiss,G., Dogan,K., & Hoy,E. (1972). Studies on the hyperactive child-VII: Neurological status compared with neurotic and normal children. *American Journal of Orthopsychiatry, 42,* 441-451.

West,D.J., & Farrington,D.P. (1973). *Who becomes delinquent? (Second Report of the Cambridge Study in Delinquent Development).* London: Heinemann.

Willerman,L. (1973). Social aspects of minimal brain dysfunction. *Annals of the New York Academy of Sciences, 205,* 164-172.

Wolff,P.H., & Hurwitz,I. (1973). Functional implications of the minimal brain damage syndrome. In S. Walzer & P.H. Wolff (Eds.), *Minimal cerebral dysfunction in children* (pp. 105-115). New York: Grune & Stratton.

Yule,W. (1973). Differential prognosis of reading backwardness and specific reading retardation. *British Journal of Educational Psychology, 43,* 244-248.

# Index